Prevention and Management of Violence: Guidance for Mental Healthcare Professionals

Prevention and Management of Violence: Guidance for Mental Healthcare Professionals

Edited by Masum Khwaja & Dominic Beer

College Report CR177
Approved by the Central Policy Committee: September 2012
Due for review: 2014

RCPsych Publications

© The Royal College of Psychiatrists 2013

RCPsych Publications is an imprint of the Royal College of Psychiatrists,
17 Belgrave Square, London SW1X 8PG
http://www.rcpsych.ac.uk

British Library Cataloguing-in-Publication Data.
A catalogue record for this book is available from the British Library.
ISBN 978-1-908020-95-6

Distributed in North America by Publishers Storage and Shipping Company.

The views presented in this book do not necessarily reflect those of the Royal College of Psychiatrists, and the publishers are not responsible for any error of omission or fact.

The Royal College of Psychiatrists is a charity registered in England and Wales (228636) and in Scotland (SC038369).

Printed by Bell & Bain Limited, Glasgow, UK.

This book is dedicated to the memory of Dominic Beer who died peacefully on 19 April 2013. He was a kind, gracious and thoughtful man, who was committed to his family, faith and profession.

Contents

Abbreviations

AMHP	approved mental health practitioner
BME	Black and minority ethnic
BNF	British National Formulary
CBT	cognitive–behavioural therapy
CCTV	closed-circuit television
CPS	Crown Prosecution Service
CTO	community treatment order
DoLS	Deprivation of Liberty Safeguards
ECG	electrocardiogram
ECHR	European Court of Human Rights
ECT	electroconvulsive therapy
EPS	extrapyramidal side-effects
GP	general practitioner
MAPPA	Multi-Agency Public Protection Arrangements
NHS	National Health Service
NICE	National Institute for Health and Care Excellence
SCT	supervised community treatment
SOAD	second opinion appointed doctor

List of boxes and tables

Working group

Joint Chair

Dominic Beer (deceased), Consultant Psychiatrist in Psychiatric Intensive Care and Challenging Behaviour, Oxleas NHS Foundation Trust, Bracton Centre, Kent

Masum Khwaja, Consultant General Adult Psychiatrist, South Westminster Mental Health Services, Central & North West London NHS Foundation Trust, and Honorary Senior Lecturer, Imperial College London

Members

Alina Bakala, Consultant Psychiatrist in Learning Disability, Central & North West London NHS Foundation Trust, The Kingswood Centre, London

Miriam Barrett, ST5, South Westminster Recovery Team, Central & North West London NHS Foundation Trust, London

Ingrid Bohnen, Consultant Psychiatrist in Learning Disability, Central & North West London NHS Foundation Trust, Westminster Learning Disability Partnership, London

Louise Butler, Professional Standards – Safeguarding Team, and Adult Safeguarding Lead, Westminster City Council, London

Ian Cumming, Consultant Forensic Psychiatrist, South London and Maudsley NHS Foundation Trust, HMP Belmarsh, London

Dominic Dougall, ST5, South Westminster Recovery Team, Central & North West London NHS Foundation Trust, London

Stephen Dye, Consultant In-Patient Psychiatrist, Norfolk and Suffolk NHS Foundation Trust, Ipswich Hospital Site, Suffolk

Laura Garrod, Forensic Nurse Specialist, Fixated Threat Assessment Centre, Barnet, Enfield & Haringey Mental Health NHS Trust, London

Hanne Jakobsen, Consultant Clinical Psychologist, South London and Maudsley NHS Foundation Trust, Maudsley Hospital, London

Douglas MacInnes, Reader in Mental Health, Centre for Health and Social Care Research, Canterbury Christ Church University, Kent

Ruth McAllister, Consultant Forensic Psychiatrist, Bracton Centre, Kent

James McIntyre, Consultant General Adult Psychiatrist, PICU and Hospital at Home, Elmleigh Hospital, Hampshire

John Olumoroti, Consultant Forensic Psychiatrist, Shaftesbury Clinic MSU, Springfield University Hospital, London

Caroline Parker, Consultant Pharmacist for Adult Mental Health Services and Lead Pharmacist for Acute Services, Independent Prescriber, Central & North West London NHS Foundation Trust, St Charles Hospital, London

Sachin Patel, ST5, South Westminster Recovery Team, Central & North West London NHS Foundation Trust, and Honorary Clinical Lecturer, Faculty of Medicine, Imperial College London

Yogesh Thakker, ST6 in Psychiatry of Learning Disability, Central & North West London NHS Foundation Trust, Riverside Centre, Hillingdon Hospital, Middlesex

Jonathan Waite, Consultant in the Psychiatry of Old Age, Nottinghamshire Healthcare NHS Trust

Anusha Wijeratne, Consultant Psychiatrist in Learning Disability, The Kingswood Centre, London

Elliot Wylde, AMHP Manager for East Hampshire, The Osborn Centre, Hampshire

Executive summary and recommendations

Organisations and individuals have a responsibility to consider how to prevent and manage aggression and violence in accordance with relevant legislation and national best practice guidelines.

There have been three previous documents produced by the Royal College of Psychiatrists on the management of violence:

1   *Strategies for the Management of Disturbed and Violent Patients in Psychiatric Units* (Council Report CR41; Royal College of Psychiatrists, 1995)
2   *Management of Imminent Violence: Clinical Practice Guidelines to Support Mental Health Services* (Occasional Paper OP41; Royal College of Psychiatrists, 1998)
3   *Good Medical Practice in the Psychiatric Care of Potentially Violent Patients in the Community* (Council Report CR80; Royal College of Psychiatrists, 2000).

In revising Council Report CR80, the Working Group amalgamated relevant aspects of the documents mentioned above, and appraised new evidence since the publication of National Institute for Health and Care Excellence (NICE) guidelines on the short-term management of disturbed/violent behaviour in psychiatric in-patient settings and emergency departments (National Institute for Health and Clinical Excellence, 2005). The revised College report provides an overview of good practice in the prevention and management of violence of patients with mental disorder.

In reflection of the multidisciplinary nature of the management of violence, membership of the Working Group tasked with producing the guidelines was itself multidisciplinary and included psychiatrists from forensic, older adult, learning disability, and general adult specialties as well as colleagues from nursing, psychology and pharmacology backgrounds.

The final document was appraised by the College's Central Policy Committee, whose membership includes carer and service user representatives.

Recommendations

1. We support the Zero Tolerance campaign against violence in the National Health Service (NHS). Organisations and individuals should not tolerate violence as an everyday, unavoidable reality of mental health services. Although incidents of violence cannot always be prevented or anticipated, a robust and considered response to incidents of violence and aggression will help to ensure a safe and more secure environment for staff, patients and carers.

2. Risk assessment is an integral component of psychiatric practice.

3. A structured clinical judgement approach to assessing the risk of violence is recommended.

4. Effective communication within the multidisciplinary team, with patients and carers, and the relevant outside agencies is an essential part of any risk management plan.

5. The assessment of risk is meaningless if no subsequent action or management plan is formulated. It is therefore necessary to consider the assessment and management of risk as one process.

6. The risk of violence cannot be removed, only minimised through effective assessment and management, and it is impossible and not always desirable to eliminate all risks. Systems of controls should not be so rigid that they stifle innovation and imaginative use of limited resources in order to achieve health benefits for service users. Responsible clinical risk-taking should be encouraged and can be described as weighing up the potential benefits and harms of exercising one choice of action over another. It involves identifying the potential risks involved (to and by a service user) and drawing up plans and actions that reflect the positive potentials and stated priorities of the service user.

7. Risks to children must be explicitly considered. If a risk to a specific child or children is identified, a referral to the appropriate child protection team must follow. Similarly, if the risk is to a vulnerable adult, the relevant adult protection policies must be followed.

8. The contribution of alcohol and substance misuse to risk must be recognised. Comorbid alcohol and substance misuse must be identified, and treatment to prevent or address alcohol and substance misuse made available.

9. By law, all hospitals in England are responsible for making sure that the care and treatment they provide meets government standards of quality and safety. Through the systematic approach of clinical governance, these standards can be met and improved alongside improving the overall care provided by organisations. In relation to the management of violence, the core elements of training and education, audit, research and development, openness, risk management and information management can be applied. These include the provision

of adequate training in risk management, ensuring processes of recording untoward incidents, transparency in reporting incidents, use of evidence-based management of violence and auditing practice to ensure basic standards are met. Through this fluid, progressive approach, organisations can provide the best quality management of violence in the clinical setting.

References

National Institute for Health and Clinical Excellence (2005) *Violence: The Short-term Management of Disturbed/Violent Behaviour in In-patient Psychiatric Settings and Emergency Departments* (Clinical Guideline CG25). NICE.

Royal College of Psychiatrists (1995) *Strategies for the Management of Disturbed and Violent Patients in Psychiatric Units* (Council Report CR41). Royal College of Psychiatrists.

Royal College of Psychiatrists (1998) *Management of Imminent Violence: Clinical Practice Guidelines to Support Mental Health Services* (Occasional Paper OP41). Royal College of Psychiatrists.

Royal College of Psychiatrists (2000) *Good Medical Practice in the Psychiatric Care of Potentially Violent Patients in the Community* (Council Report CR80). Royal College of Psychiatrists.

CHAPTER 1

Legislation relevant to the management of violence by persons with mental disorders

Dominic Dougall and John Olumoroti

This chapter provides an overview of the legislative frameworks that are relevant to the management of violence by persons with mental disorders in the UK. As three jurisdictions apply (England and Wales, Scotland, and Northern Ireland), individual frameworks and their variants are not discussed in detail. Rather, substantial differences relevant to the management of violence are highlighted. Professionals should refer to the respective frameworks for detailed guidance.

Management of violence refers not only to acute episodes, but also to the prevention or reduction of the risk of future violence. The core principles guiding routine medical practice of 'consent' and 'do no harm' remain relevant. Legislation provides a framework when coercion may be necessary to manage an acute violent act, manage the immediate risk of further violence or manage longer-term risk of violence.

Three strands of legislation are relevant to this report: the Human Rights Act 1998, mental health acts and mental capacity acts. The Human Rights Act applies to all three jurisdictions. The Mental Capacity Act 2005 and the Mental Health Act 1983 apply to England and Wales. Scotland is covered by the Mental Health (Care and Treatment) (Scotland) Act 2003 and the Adults with Incapacity (Scotland) Act 2000. Mental health legislation in Northern Ireland comprises the Mental Health (Amendment) (Northern Ireland) Order 2004. In certain circumstances, common law 'duty of care' may also be relied on, which remains necessary in Northern Ireland and which does not yet have an equivalent to the Mental Capacity Act.

Human Rights Act 1998

Compliance with the Human Rights Act is required when a function is of a public nature. The Act requires public authorities to act in accordance with the European Convention on Human Rights and the European Court of Human Rights (ECHR) which came into force in 1953. The Act would, for example, apply to the NHS and local authorities. It recognises certain rights and freedoms, with the ECHR hearing alleged breaches. The Act serves to allow UK citizens to seek redress in the UK regarding possible contraventions without having to apply immediately to the ECHR.

The Human Rights Act includes the notion of proportionality, which is highly relevant in the management of violence. It recognises that on occasions it may be necessary to restrict someone's rights, but any restriction must be kept to the minimum necessary to achieve the required objective.

Articles 2, 3, 5 and 8 are most relevant to this report and are described in more detail. Article 6 relates to the provision of the Mental Health Act, but less so violence; however, it does state that everyone has the 'right to a fair trial' in relation to both civil rights and criminal charges. The tribunal or court should be independent and impartial. The remaining articles are less relevant.

Article 2: Right to life

Article 2 states that 'Everyone's right to life shall be protected by law' and 'Deprivation of life shall not be regarded as inflicted in contravention of this article when it results from the use of force which is no more than absolutely necessary:

(a) in defence of any person from unlawful violence
(b) in order to effect a lawful arrest or to prevent the escape of a person lawfully detained
(c) in action lawfully taken for the purpose of quelling a riot or insurrection.'

It has been held that Article 2 implies 'in certain well defined circumstances a positive obligation on the authorities to take preventive operational measures to protect an individual whose life is at risk from the criminal acts of another individual' (*Osman v. United Kingdom* [2000]).

The work of public authorities may be affected by Article 2 in a variety of ways. A public authority with knowledge of the 'existence of a real and immediate risk to someone's life from the criminal acts of another individual' should act to protect that person. A public authority should ensure those in its care are safe. If 'planning an operation which may result in a risk to life', then 'the minimum necessary force' must be used. If working with 'persons known to be dangerous', then steps should be taken to protect public safety (Ministry of Justice, 2006).

Article 3: Prohibition of torture

Article 3 states that 'no one shall be subjected to torture or to inhuman or degrading treatment or punishment'. Measures need to be taken to ensure this does not occur in psychiatric hospitals where individuals are potentially more vulnerable. The exact scope of this article has been regularly considered by the ECHR, which has found that 'compulsory treatment is capable of being inhuman treatment (or in extreme cases even torture) contrary to Article 3, if its effect on the person concerned reaches a sufficient level of severity'. But that 'a measure which is convincingly shown to be of therapeutic necessity from the point of view of established principles of medicine cannot in principle be regarded as inhuman and degrading' (*Herczegfalvy v. Austria* [1993]).

Article 5: Right to liberty and security

Article 5 states that everyone has the right not to be 'arrested or detained' apart from exceptions such as 'the lawful detention of a person after conviction by a competent court' and 'persons of unsound mind'. Lawful detention in relation to persons of unsound mind would more likely be under the auspices of the Mental Health Act, although circumstances may occur where detention under the Mental Capacity Act or, in limited circumstances, under common law 'best interests' is necessary.

Article 8: Right to respect for private and family life

Although everyone has the right to private and family life and their correspondence, certain restrictions exist. Relevant exclusions include public safety, prevention of crime, protection of health or morals and the protection of rights and freedoms of others. Compulsory administration of treatment would infringe Article 8 unless it is covered by law, such as the Mental Health Act. Such treatment would need to be proportionate and legitimate, such as reducing the risk associated with a person's mental disorder and improving their health (Department of Health, 2008).

Mental Capacity Act 2005

England & Wales

The Mental Capacity Act 2005 provides a statutory framework for professionals and others who care for people with impaired capacity. Any action resulting from the use of the Act must be assessed as being in the person's best interests (*Herczegfalvy v. Austria* [1993]). Consideration must also be given as to whether the decision can be deferred until the person regains capacity. It is important to recognise when the Act may be indicated or when the Mental Health Act is more appropriate: a patient with a mental disorder who lacks capacity to consent to treatment in a psychiatric hospital is liable to be detained under the Mental Health Act rather than receive treatment under the Mental Capacity Act (Department for Constitutional Affairs, 2007).

In relation to the management of violence, the Mental Capacity Act *Code of Practice* attempts to make clear the nature of restraint that is acceptable. Section 6 of the Act provides authority to restrain a person who lacks capacity. Restraint is defined as: (1) 'the use, or the threat of the use of force against a person who resists the action'; and (2) 'restricts a person's liberty of movement, whether or not the person resists'. Two conditions are applied to the use of restraint: (1) 'to reasonably believe that it is necessary to prevent harm to a person' and (2) 'that it is a proportionate response to the likelihood of the person suffering harm and the seriousness of that harm' (Department for Constitutional Affairs, 2007). In addition, the *Code of Practice* describes circumstances where the Mental Capacity Act may be relevant in the prevention of violence: 'a person may also be at risk of harm if they behave in a way that encourages others to assault or exploit them (for example, by behaving in a dangerously provocative way)' (p. 107).

Restraining a person who is likely to cause harm but is not at risk of suffering harm themselves appears not to be covered by the Mental Capacity Act. Any such action would have to be justified in terms of the professional's duty of care to the person at risk of suffering harm, and may need to be managed under common law.

If restraint is used frequently, this may amount to a deprivation of liberty. This is not covered by Section 6, and if a patient in a hospital or a resident in a care home is at risk of deprivation of liberty, authorisation should be sought under the Deprivation of Liberty Safeguards (DoLS) from the appropriate supervisory body. It should be noted that DoLS cannot normally be used for a patient in hospital if the necessary care or treatment consists in whole or in part of the medical treatment for a mental disorder (Department of Health, 2005).

Under the provisions of 'advance decisions to refuse treatment' (Sections 24–26), it is possible to make an advance decision to refuse any specified medical treatment – this might include medication for the management of potential violence (Department for Constitutional Affairs, 2007). Medication given under Part IV of the Mental Health Act is not covered by these provisions.

Scotland

Adults with Incapacity (Scotland) Act 2000

This is broadly similar to the Mental Capacity Act. Guidance specific to violence is found in Section 47(7). This states that the use of force or detention is not authorised unless it is immediately necessary. The use of force or detention should only be for as long as is necessary and be consistent with a decision that may be made by a competent court. The Act should not be used to treat a patient for a mental disorder in hospital against their will.

Northern Ireland

To date, equivalent legislation has not been introduced in Northern Ireland.

Mental Health Act 1983

England & Wales

The potential for a mental health service user to imminently be responsible for acts of violence is frequently the reason for seeking detention under the Mental Health Act. It is recognised that: 'Where a patient has been detained under the [Mental Health Act], there is an implied right for staff to exercise a degree of control over the activities of the patient' (*Pountney v. Griffiths* [1976]).

When detaining a person under the Mental Health Act, appropriate medical treatment needs to be available, as defined by Section 145(1) of the Act, and paragraph 6.2 of the *Code of Practice* (Department of Health, 2008). The *Code of Practice* states that medical treatment also includes interventions other than medication. This may consist of nursing treatment only, which could include restraint.

In the statute, specific reference to violence is made in two places in relation to emergency treatment. Section 62 authorises treatment which is immediately necessary and of minimum interference to prevent a 'patient from behaving violently or being a danger to himself or to others'. In Section 64C there is provision for treatment which would normally require either consent from the patient or authorisation from a second opinion appointed doctor (SOAD) in certain circumstances where the treatment 'is immediately necessary, represents the minimum interference necessary to prevent the patient from behaving violently or being a danger to himself or to others and is not irreversible or hazardous'.

The *Code of Practice* contains extensive guidance on responses to violence, principally in Chapter 15 'Safe and therapeutic responses to disturbed behaviour' (Department of Health, 2008). Recommendations include suitable assessment for potential risk of violence, identification of warning signs, de-escalation, control and restraint, and seclusion policies.

Community treatment orders

Supervised community treatment (SCT) was introduced in England and Wales in November 2008. Under SCT, patients who have been detained in hospital for treatment under Section 3 and unrestricted Part III (forensic) patients will, on discharge, become subject to a community treatment order (CTO), requiring them to comply with certain conditions. Patients have to be considered for SCT if they are receiving more than 7 days of home leave under Section 17. Supervised community treatment can only be imposed on patients directly following a period of compulsory detention in hospital.

Patients with mental disorders who do not continue with their treatment (in particular, their medication) when they are discharged from hospital may, if their mental health deteriorates, become a danger either to themselves or to other people, and eventually have to be compulsorily readmitted to hospital. The aim of SCT is to maintain stability and reduce the risk of relapse through the use of conditions that ensure the patient receives necessary treatment. Supervised community treatment allows for recall to a designated hospital. This may allow risks associated with relapse, such as violence, to be more effectively managed and reduced through earlier readmission. Ideally, the conditions of the CTO will have prevented a relapse in the first case. The use of SCT is further described in Chapter 25 of the *Code of Practice* (Department of Health, 2008).

Before the advent of SCT, the Mental Health Act included various powers to manage patients by compulsion in the community and these included guardianship (Sections 7 and 37), supervised aftercare (Section 25) and leave of absence (Section 17). Of these, guardianship remains relevant (with Section 17 used only for short-term leave) and enables patients to receive care in the community where it cannot be provided by the use of compulsory powers (Department of Health, 2008). The powers of a guardian (who may be a local authority or a named private individual) may include requiring a person to live at a specified address, to attend for treatment at a specified place and allow health professionals access to their home. However, unless the patient consents, treatment cannot be imposed. Further, the guardian does not have powers to use force to make a patient attend for treatment or to enter their home.

Community treatment orders have been in place for some years in the USA, Canada, Australia and New Zealand and were introduced into Scotland in October 2005. The difficulty in predicting a risk incident has been acknowledged. The benefits of CTOs have long been questioned (Moncrieff & Smyth, 1999). It has also been suggested that thousands of people may have to be placed under compulsion in the community to prevent one homicide (Crawford, 2000; Szmukler, 2000).

There have been a number of reviews of the effectiveness of CTO systems across the world, although research is limited and patchy and many reviews are subject to methodological limitations (Atkinson *et al*, 2005; Churchill, 2007). A Cochrane review of two randomised controlled trials in the USA found little evidence to indicate that compulsory community treatment was effective in any of the main outcome indices: health service use, readmission to hospital, social functioning, arrests, mental state, quality of life, homelessness or satisfaction with care (Kisely *et al*, 2005). People receiving compulsory community treatment were, however, less likely to be victims of violent or non-violent crime (Churchill, 2007). A retrospective case-note review suggested that CTOs halved the number of episodes of aggression (Ingram *et al*, 2009).

One relevant question that has been asked is what impact will SCT have on homicides by people with a mental illness? There is no reliable way of calculating exactly how many homicides might be prevented by a CTO. There has been no discernible reduction in the overall rates of homicides by people with a mental illness in Canada, Australia or New Zealand as a result of CTOs having been in place for some years. In England, independent inquiries into cases of homicide committed by those who have been in contact with the psychiatric service, mandatory since 1994, have commonly cited non-adherence to medication as one factor leading to the incident (National Confidential Inquiry into Suicide and Homicide by People with Mental Illness, 2006). In such cases it is possible that had the individual been under SCT they may have adhered to their treatment regime, potentially averting a homicide.

Restriction orders

Restriction orders (such as Section 41) may be imposed by a Crown Court alongside a hospital order (e.g. Section 37) if the court thinks it necessary for protecting the public from harm. Restriction orders can last indefinitely and require consent from the Secretary of State for Justice to approve aspects of management such as discharge from hospital and the approval of community placement. Although the order may be indefinite, it may be lifted by the Secretary of State when the order is no longer considered necessary for the protection of others.

Scotland

Mental Health (Care and Treatment) (Scotland) Act 2003

The key differences between this Act and the Mental Health Act have previously been described (Zigmond, 2008). These relate to capacity, compulsion for more than 28 days, and responsibilities of practitioners, of which capacity is most relevant to this report. Scottish legislation does not allow compulsion when a person retains capacity, whereas the Mental Health Act will allow compulsion when there is risk to the safety of others (as well as risks to self and health), even when capacity is retained.

Northern Ireland

Mental Health (Amendment) (Northern Ireland) Order 2004

Legislation in Northern Ireland does not provide for the use of CTOs; it is otherwise not substantially different to the Mental Health Act.

Indeterminate sentences for public protection

This legislation is not specific to mental health patients, but it may be applied to offenders with a mental health disorder. The sentence of Imprisonment for Public Protection was created by the Criminal Justice Act 2003 and implemented in April 2005. It is issued to those offenders who are seen by the courts as dangerous but who do not require a life sentence. Similar to a life sentence, prisoners are given a tariff or minimum term which they must serve before being considered for release. After release they are subject to recall if they breach the terms of their licence. Similar arrangements were legislated for in Northern Ireland by the Criminal Justice (Northern Ireland) Order 2008.

References

Atkinson, J. M., Reilly, R., Garner, H. C., *et al* (2005) *Review of Literature Relating to Mental Health Legislation*. Scottish Executive.

Churchill, R. (2007) *International Experiences of using Community Treatment Orders*. Department of Health.

Crawford, M. (2000) Homicide is impossible to predict. *Psychiatric Bulletin*, **24**, 152.

Department for Constitutional Affairs (2007) *Mental Capacity Act 2005: Code of Practice*. TSO (The Stationery Office).

Department of Health (2005) *Deprivation of Liberty Safeguards: Code of Practice to Supplement the Main Mental Capacity Act 2005 Code of Practice*. TSO (The Stationery Office).

Department of Health (2008) *Code of Practice: Mental Health Act 1983*. TSO (The Stationery Office.

Ingram, G., Muirhead, D. & Harvey, C. (2009) Effectiveness of community treatment orders for treatment of schizophrenia with oral or depot antipsychotic medication: changes in problem behaviours and social functioning. *Australian and New Zealand Journal of Psychiatry*, **43**, 1077–1083.

Kisely, S., Campbell, L. A. & Preston, N. (2005) *Compulsory Community and Involuntary Outpatient Treatment for People with Severe Mental Disorders (Review)*. Wiley.

Ministry of Justice (2006) *Human Rights: Human Lives. A Handbook for Public Authorities*. TSO (The Stationery Office).

Moncrieff, J. & Smyth, M. (1999) Community treatment orders – a bridge too far? *Psychiatric Bulletin*, **23**, 644–646.

National Confidential Inquiry into Suicide and Homicide by People with Mental Illness (2006) *Avoidable Deaths: Five Year Report of the National Confidential Inquiry into Suicide and Homicide by People with a Mental Illness*. National Confidential Inquiry into Suicide and Homicide by People with Mental Illness.

Szmukler, G. (2000) Homicide inquiries. What sense do they make? *Psychiatric Bulletin*, **24**, 6–10.

Zigmond, T. (2008) Changing mental health legislation in the UK. *Advances in Psychiatric Treatment*, **14**, 81–83.

Herczegfalvy v. Austria [1993] 15 EHRR 437.
Osman v. United Kingdom [2000] 29 ECHR 245.
Pountney v. Griffiths [1976] AC 314.

CHAPTER 2

Safeguarding vulnerable adults and children exposed to violence

Louise Butler, Masum Khwaja and Miriam Barrett

The vulnerability of adults with mental illness to violence has been highlighted by a recent meta-analysis which included 21 studies reporting violence prevalence estimates against adults with disabilities (mainly 18 years and older) from 1990 to 2010 (Hughes *et al*, 2012). The study showed that the odds of a person with mental illness experiencing physical, sexual or domestic violence was almost four times higher than for adults without any disabilities. In fact, people with mental illness are ten times more likely to be victims than perpetrators of violence. One of the reasons for the particular vulnerability of people with mental illness may be the interpersonal difficulties inherent to those conditions. Other contributing factors seem to be the need for personal assistance in daily living, reduced physical and emotional defences, social stigma, discrimination, communication barriers and exclusion from education and employment.

In the UK, about 17000 children and young people live with a parent who has a severe and enduring mental illness, and about 175 000 children care for a parent or other family member with a mental disorder (Mental Health Foundation, 2013). Some of these children may experience increased levels of emotional, psychological and behavioural problems. Reasons for this include:

- inherited genes that may make them more vulnerable to mental ill health
- the child's environment (e.g. parents with a severe illness are more likely to live in poverty)
- the child's situation (e.g. feeling insecure/anxious that their parent will become unwell)
- the stigma attached to living with a parent with mental illness (e.g. being bullied at school).

In addition, children may not ask for help because of the fear that they will be taken away from their parent(s).

In light of the increasing evidence base, government policy on the safeguarding of vulnerable adults and children has continued to evolve over the past decade. Services and professionals have a duty to safeguard vulnerable adults who are at risk of violence or of being exposed to violence, and the risk to children must be explicitly considered in all cases.

Safeguarding adults

The government White Paper *Equity and Excellence* (Department of Health, 2010a) makes clear that patients must be at the heart of the NHS.

Safeguarding adults is relevant to the NHS, as services are accountable to patients for their safety and well-being as well as delivering high-quality care. Some patients may be unable to uphold their rights and protect themselves from harm or abuse. They may have the greatest dependency and yet be unable to hold the service to account for the quality of care they receive.

A key safeguarding document on a national framework of standards for good practice and outcomes in adult protection work describes a range of activities that focus on those patients who are least able to protect themselves from harm (Association of Directors of Adult Social Services, 2005). It covers a spectrum of activity aimed at:

- preventing safeguarding concerns arising through provision of high-quality care
- providing effective responses where harm or abuse occurs, supporting the patient's choices through multi-agency safeguarding adults procedures.

Local authorities have the lead role in coordinating the multi-agency approach to safeguarding adults at risk from abuse. In addition to the strategic role of the local authority, there will be different local arrangements for each borough to deliver safeguarding responses to concerns that an adult at risk is being abused, in line with local policy and procedures. The local authority should:

- ensure that any adult's concern is acted on in line with relevant policy and procedures;
- coordinate the actions that relevant organisations take in accordance with their own duties and responsibilities. This does not mean that local authorities undertake all activities: relevant organisations have their own roles and responsibilities. Further guidance on legal interface issues can be sought in the recent publication *Safeguarding Adults at Risk of Harm* (Social Care Institute for Excellence, 2011);
- ensure a continued focus on the adult at risk and due consideration to other adults or children;
- ensure that key decisions are made to an agreed timescale;
- ensure that an interim and a final protection plan are put in place with adequate arrangements for review and monitoring;

- ensure that actions leading from investigation are proportionate to the level of the risk and enable the adult at risk to be in control unless there are clear, recorded reasons why this should not be the case;
- ensure independent scrutiny of circumstances leading to the concern for an adult and to safeguarding adult work (Department of Health, 2006);
- facilitate learning the lessons from practice and communicate these to the relevant boards (Department of Health, 2010b).

Safeguarding children

Safeguarding children may be defined as the process of protecting children from abuse or neglect, preventing impairment of their health and development, and ensuring they are growing up in circumstances consistent with the provision of safe and effective care that enables them to have optimum life chances and enter adulthood successfully.

The impact on children who have been exposed to violence is similar to the effects of any other abuse or trauma and will depend on factors such as the severity and nature of violence, the duration of exposure to violence, the child's gender, age, disability, socioeconomic and cultural background, and the presence and quality of emotional support of family members.

There may be an increased risk of physical injury during an incident, either by accident or because the child may, for example, attempt to intervene in incidents of domestic violence between parents. Even when not directly injured, children may be distressed by witnessing the physical and emotional suffering of a parent. Exposure to parental conflict, even when violence is not present, may arouse distressing feelings in a child such as anxiety, fear, sadness, loneliness, helplessness and despair, which may be associated with deterioration in educational achievement or maladaptive behaviours such as social withdrawal, and aggressive, antisocial or criminal behaviour deterioration (Onyskiw, 2003; Cleaver et al, 2010).

Protecting children from harm and promoting their welfare is dependent on a shared responsibility between individual practitioners, supported by the commitment of senior managers to safeguard children and by ensuring there are clear lines of accountability.

The Children Act 2004 established the formation of multi-agency local safeguarding children boards. These consist of representatives from local partner agencies such as housing, health, police and probation services. The boards are charged with coordinating the functions of all partner agencies in relation to safeguarding children.

The document *Working Together to Safeguard Children* (Department for Children, Schools and Families, 2010) sets out how organisations and individuals should work together to safeguard and promote the welfare of children and young people in accordance with the Children Act 1989 and the Children Act 2004.

References

Association of Directors of Adult Social Services (2005) *Safeguarding Adults: A National Framework of Standards for Good Practice and Outcomes in Adult Protection Work*. ADASS.

Cleaver, H., Unell, I. & Aldgate, A. (2010) *Children's Needs – Parenting Capacity: The Impact of Parental Mental Illness, Learning Disability, Problem Alcohol and Drug Use, and Domestic Violence on Children's Safety and Development (2nd edn)*. TSO (The Stationery Office).

Department for Children, Schools and Families (2010) *Working Together to Safeguard Children: A Guide to Interagency Working to Safeguard and Promote the Welfare of Children*. HM Government.

Department of Health (2006) *Memorandum of Understanding: Investigating Patient Safety Incidents Involving Unexpected Death or Serious Untoward Harm*. Department of Health.

Department of Health (2010a) *Equity and Excellence: Liberating the NHS* (White Paper). Department of Health.

Department of Health (2010b) *Clinical Governance and Adult Safeguarding: An Integrated Process*. Department of Health.

Hughes, K., Bellis, M. A., Jones, L., *et al* (2012) Prevalence and risk of violence against adults with disabilities: a systematic review and meta-analysis of observational studies. *Lancet*, **379**, 1621–1629.

Mental Health Foundation (2013) Parents. Mental Health Foundation (http://www.mentalhealth.org.uk/help-information/mental-health-a-z/P/parents/).

Onyskiw, J. E. (2003) Domestic violence and children's adjustment: a review of research. *Journal of Emotional Abuse*, **3**, 11–45.

Social Care Institute for Excellence (2011) *Safeguarding Adults at Risk of Harm: A Legal Guide for Practitioners*. SCIE.

CHAPTER 3

Risk assessment and management

Ruth McAllister and Sachin Patel

Risk assessment forms an integral part of psychiatric practice. It covers a wide range of potential harms to which patients may be exposed, or which they may pose to themselves or others. Risk assessment may be defined as the systematic collection of information from all available sources to estimate the degree to which harm (to self or others) is likely at some point in time (O'Rourke & Bird, 2001). It begins at first contact with a patient and needs to be reviewed regularly in light of changing circumstances and new information; it is a dynamic process. Risk assessment is meaningless, however, unless it is linked with a management plan which aims to reduce the likelihood that harm will occur, or to reduce its severity if it does occur. Risk assessment and management should be an integrated process.

In the past 20 years the concept of 'dangerousness' has been left behind as it is increasingly recognised that risk to others is not a trait inherent in a patient, but the product of a range of interacting factors. Some of these factors are patient-related; some are related to the people around the patient, some to the environment and some to chance. When a mental health professional recognises a significant risk of violence, they are under a professional obligation to take steps to manage and reduce it by all practicable means (Department of Health, 2008).

There is, however, a danger in adopting an overly risk-oriented and risk-averse approach to mental healthcare. The association between certain mental disorders and violent behaviour is established; however, the spectrum of risk and the relative rarity of the most serious violence must also be considered (National Confidential Inquiry into Suicide and Homicide by People with Mental Illness, 2011). A Royal College of Psychiatrists' briefing document offers a helpful commentary on moving beyond a 'culture of blame' (Morgan, 2007).

In this chapter, we outline current views on the principles of assessing and managing the risk of violence, as well as some of the practical implications. This is not intended to be exhaustive and readers are encouraged to refer to the publications cited for further guidance.

Principles of risk assessment and management

An important principle in risk management is that it should be positive – it should involve improving the service user's quality of life and plans for recovery (Department of Health, 2007; Royal College of Psychiatrists, 2008). There is a danger that preoccupation with risk will lead to defensive practice, which may in itself become a risk factor for negative outcomes if it damages the therapeutic alliance, leads to unwarranted restrictions being placed on the person's autonomy or increases social exclusion.

The College's report *Rethinking Risk to Others in Mental Health Services* (Royal College of Psychiatrists, 2008) sets out the general principles listed below.

- Accurate risk prediction is never possible at an individual level. Nevertheless, the use of structured risk assessment when systematically applied by a clinical team within a tiered approach to risk assessment can enhance clinical judgement. This will contribute to effective and safe service delivery.
- Risk assessment is a vital element in the process of clinical assessment. It enables psychiatrists to reach a reasoned judgement on the level and type of risk factors for violence present in an individual case. This facilitates clinical interventions for those risk factors amenable to clinical treatment within the resources available to a clinical team.
- Risk assessment informs risk management and there should be a direct follow-through from assessment to management.
- The best quality of care can be provided only if there are established links between the needs assessments of service users and risk assessment.
- Positive risk management is part of a carefully constructed plan and is a required competence for all mental health practitioners.
- Risk management must recognise and promote the patient's strengths and should support recovery.
- Risk management requires an organisational strategy as well as competent efforts by individual practitioners.
- Risk management needs to recognise the role of other agencies.

The Department of Health's (2007) report *Best Practice in Managing Risk* provides an essential review of the fundamentals, principles and practice of managing risk and an overview of risk factors for violence.

Approaches to assessing and managing risk

Risk assessment may be clinical (based on the history, mental state and knowledge of the patient's circumstances), actuarial (using statistical approaches to measuring risk based on population studies) or a combination of both, known as structured clinical judgement. In this approach, clinical details are organised systematically and given weightings derived from actuarial studies.

This is a helpful basis for risk management plans, since factors relevant to the risk of violence are considered systematically, formulated explicitly and communicated in a clearly intelligible format. Information from all possible collateral sources should be included, with particular emphasis on informant accounts from relatives and other close contacts of the patient.

The risk management plan should include consideration of the type of violence which is to be anticipated, the likely victims, exacerbating and alleviating factors, and the duration and immediacy of any risk. The views of the patient and carer should be included: patients should be encouraged to contribute to management plans and express preferences. They should be supported in making advance directives, where appropriate, on how they would like their behaviour to be managed in future if they become disturbed.

Standardised risk assessment tools contribute to a thorough understanding of the present situation and the anticipation of risks in the short term, but for an individual they cannot be predictive. A helpful appraisal of many of the violence risk assessment tools available is included in the Department of Health's guidelines on best practice in managing risk (Department of Health, 2007).

Risk assessment at a local level

Most NHS trusts have some form of clinical risk assessment in place but, until recently, there has been little attempt to validate them. The most basic approach used in general psychiatric settings involves ticking boxes relating to a patient's history and may offer a false sense of reassurance (Royal College of Psychiatrists, 2008). In 2006, the independent inquiry into the care and treatment of John Barrett (South West London Strategic Health Authority, 2006) recommended that the Department of Health should consider the establishment of common risk assessment standards for secure units. The Royal College of Psychiatrists went further and recommended the development of a standardised approach throughout mental health services (Royal College of Psychiatrists, 2008). Box 3.1 (p. 16) summarises the relevant recommendations.

Multi-agency working

Liaison with other agencies, such as the police and Social Services, may be a necessary part of information-gathering, which enables a thorough assessment of risk. Effective communication between relevant agencies is also vital when implementing a risk management plan.

The content of discharge letters to general practitioners (GPs), copied to patients and carers (as agreed), must include: details of risk to self or others; diagnosis; treatment; indicators of relapse; and the details of any agreed risk management plan (Royal College of Psychiatrists, 2008).

Box 3.1 Recommendations for risk assessment

- Risk assessment forms should be evidence based. Mental health trusts and boards should ensure that all risk assessment forms in use in the organisation are validated for use with each specific patient group and reflect the current evidence base.
- A national standard approach is required to risk assessment. A standard approach to risk assessment should be developed throughout all mental health services nationally, with adaptation to suit different patient groups. The College recommends that the [National Institute for Health and Care Excellence] (NICE) and SIGN Health give consideration to the development of specific guidelines on the management of risk to others.
- Quality improvement networks should include risk assessment. The College Centre for Quality Improvement (CCQI) should consider the feasibility of incorporating structured risk assessment into all quality improvement networks. The Risk Management Authority in Scotland has developed 'traffic light' indicators for assessment tools, which will inform practice in Scotland, and these could be developed for use in the rest of the UK.

Royal College of Psychiatrists (2008: p. 39)

As discussed in Chapter 2, the risks to children must be explicitly considered. If a risk to a specific child or children is identified, a referral to the appropriate child protection team must follow. Similarly, if the risk is to a vulnerable adult, the relevant adult protection policies must be followed.

Referral for specialist forensic risk assessment may be helpful.

Liaison with the police and Crown Prosecution Service is considered in Chapter 11. Where a significant risk to others has been identified, referral to the local multi-agency public protection panel should also be considered (see Chapter 11).

Working collaboratively with carers and service users

Risk assessment should be conducted collaboratively between mental health services, the service user and carers, in a way that is as trusting as possible. Service users' experiences and views of their level of risk and their personal risk 'triggers' should be fully considered, and the role of families and carers in keeping a service user safe acknowledged (Royal College of Psychiatrists, 2008).

Summary

- Risk assessment is an integral component of psychiatric practice.
- The risk of violence cannot be removed, only minimised through effective assessment and management.

- Risk management must involve careful consideration of the potential benefits and harms of the planned interventions, taking into account the needs of the service user and of others who may be at risk.
- A structured clinical judgement approach to assessing the risk of violence is recommended.
- Local risk assessment and management procedures should be informed by national guidance and trusts should work with the relevant quality networks to develop a standardised approach.
- Effective communication within the multidisciplinary team, with the patient and carers and with the relevant outside agencies is an essential part of any risk management plan.

Further reading

Buchanan, A. (2008) Risk of violence by psychiatric patients: beyond the 'actuarial versus clinical' assessment debate. *Psychiatric Services*, **59**, 184–190.

Singh, J. P., Grann, M. & Fazel, S. (2011) A comparative study of violence risk assessment tools: A systematic review and meta regression analysis of 68 studies involving 25,980 participants. *Clinical Psychology Review*, **31**, 499–513.

Webster, C. D., Douglas, K. S., Eaves, D., *et al* (1997) *HCR-20: Assessing Risk for Violence (Version 2)*. Mental Health, Law, and Policy Institute, Simon Fraser University.

References

Department of Health (2007) *Best Practice in Managing Risk: Principles and Guidance for Best Practice in the Assessment and Management of Risk to Self and Others in Mental Health Services.* Department of Health.

Department of Health (2008) *Code of Practice: Mental Health Act 1983.* TSO (The Stationery Office).

Morgan, J. F. (2007) *'Giving up the Culture of Blame': Risk Assessment and Risk Management in Psychiatric Practice.* Royal College of Psychiatrists.

National Confidential Inquiry into Suicide and Homicide by People with Mental Illness (2011) *Annual Report: England and Wales.* University of Manchester.

O'Rourke, M. & Bird, L. (2001) *Risk Management in Mental Health: A Practical Guide to Individual Care and Community Safety.* Mental Health Foundation.

Royal College of Psychiatrists (2008) *Rethinking Risk to Others in Mental Health Services* (College Report CR150). Royal College of Psychiatrists.

South West London Strategic Health Authority (2006) *Report of the Independent Inquiry into the Care and Treatment of John Barrett.* NHS London.

CHAPTER 4

Risk prevention and non-pharmacological management of violence in acute settings

Sachin Patel, Douglas MacInnes, John Olumoroti and Ruth McAllister

When the Zero Tolerance campaign against violence in the NHS was launched in 1999, very few people thought it would relate to mental health services. However, the campaign was timely and coincided in a movement towards not accepting violence as an everyday, unavoidable reality of mental health services. This change in values has seen an increase in the belief that more can and should be done to reduce the rates of violence and aggression. Although services may not be able to stop or anticipate all incidents of violence, they certainly should not tolerate violent behaviour.

In addition, we would reiterate that effective risk assessment and management prior to imminent violence is vital in prevention. Evidence from randomised controlled trials is emerging, showing that aggressive incidents can be reduced significantly through structured risk assessment (van de Sande *et al*, 2011; Abderhalden *et al*, 2008).

Prevention of violence

Containment v. engagement

Traditional thinking has often included the notion that increasing containment interventions by staff and restrictive regimes produces safer environments and decreases disturbance. In contrast to this logic, Bowers *et al* (2006) in a multicentre study in several European cities found that the delivery of 'containment' interventions by staff did not produce a proportional reduction in disturbance. Positive engagement over observation and activity over boredom are being increasingly recognised as highly effective concepts in producing dramatically reduced levels of aggression.

Any successful method of engagement over containment needs to include a strong emphasis on a programme of structured activity in conjunction with an appropriate risk assessment. This should be delivered in a consistent fashion and facilitated both on and away from the ward environment. Successful interaction and positive engagement within a framework and in a setting that allows for safe observation are key characteristics central to reducing violent incidents.

Ward regimes

In 1999, the Standing Nursing and Midwifery Advisory Committee produced a report in response to published and damming accounts of boredom and inactivity in mental health in-patient hospitals, and gave persuasive accounts of how this is related to disturbance. Subsequent guidance from NICE, the Royal College of Psychiatrists, the Department of Health and Star Wards has recommended the provision of recovery-focused meaningful activity in mental health in-patient settings (Department of Health, 2001; National Institute for Health and Clinical Excellence, 2005; Janner, 2006; Cresswell & Beavon, 2010).

A structured and system-wide approach to provision of meaningful activity should be represented by the development of a daily programme available to all service users whose care plan, risk assessment and legal status provide opportunity for this (Janner, 2006; Cresswell & Beavon, 2010). Hospital therapy departments should be central to the development, administration and logistical management of such programmes. The programme contents should be distributed to and displayed within wards. All ward-based staff should be prepared to support the programme by encouraging and enabling service users to engage in it, while providing a range of social, recreational and therapeutic activities.

Standard operating procedures for leave

The value of escorted and unescorted leave is a well-accepted strategy for reducing tension and potential escalation towards violence. Leave should be supported by adequate staffing, risk management and standard operating procedures. The use of mobile communications and a standard operational policy can be defined. Dix *et al* (2008) suggest a number of procedural steps and measures to facilitate such an approach.

- Prior to commencing escorted leave, staff should check that they have access to an agreed method of communication such as a two-way radio or mobile telephone. The escorting staff should check the device is working before departure and ensure the shift coordinator is aware of their expected time of return.
- If there is a deviation from the stated plan or expected duration of leave, the escort will inform the unit.

Standard operational policy should also recommend action to take if the service user becomes disturbed or attempts to leave the escort. This includes:

- attempting verbal negotiation
- failing this, contacting the unit and assessing the appropriateness of physical intervention
- only attempting physical intervention if safe to do so
- if physical intervention is inappropriate, following the service user at a safe distance, contacting the other staff by radio with situation reports at 5-minute intervals.

Interpersonal relationships and the use of self

Another important area in the prevention of violence and skill development among mental health staff is the use of 'self' within the context of trusting relationships as a means of de-escalation of disturbance. Relational security is the knowledge and understanding staff have of a patient, the environment in which care is provided, and the translation of that information into appropriate responses and engagement and care. Relational security is not simply about having 'a good relationship' with a patient. Safe and effective relationships between staff and patients must be professional, therapeutic and purposeful, with understood limits. Limits enable staff to maintain their professional integrity and say 'no'.

Substance misuse and environmental searches

Substance misuse is a known risk factor for violence and acute intoxication or withdrawal states can contribute significantly to the onset of violence. On healthcare premises, appropriately trained members of staff are entitled to undertake lawful searches of patients, visitors and their belongings with their consent. The Mental Health Act 1983 *Code of Practice* (Department of Health, 2008) details the legislation regarding conducting searches in the hospital setting for those consenting and also not consenting to searches. In order to be justified, there must be reason to believe that the search could detect and prevent a risk of harm to the patient or others, and the search must be proportionate to the risk. This applies, for example, on units where there is a suspicion of illicit drug use which exacerbates the risk of disturbed and violent behaviour.

Healthcare staff are not entitled to undertake intimate body searches and are not as expert as the police in carrying out environmental searches. In units where the risks are high, consideration should be given to reporting any evidence of criminal activity, such as illicit drug dealing, to the police. This is clearly a serious step which requires cooperation and support from the healthcare team for both patients and police. The intrusion needs to be balanced against the potential risks and the necessity to protect vulnerable patients as well as staff from serious harm.

Healthcare trusts should have a local policy on personal and environmental searches. It should explicitly set out measures to be taken to protect the patient's dignity. It should specify the action to be taken when consent for searching is denied. The policy should also include the actions to be taken if a search uncovers evidence of criminal activity. Protocols should be developed, in liaison with the local police, for recording, storing and handing over evidence to the police.

Where substance misuse is a factor in the risk of violence, it may be helpful to include drug testing as part of the management plan. Testing may help to elucidate the relationship between intoxication and fluctuations in mental state; it may provide a therapeutic boundary to help some patients to maintain abstinence, as it may provide corroboration of abstinence or suspected relapse, particularly for patients in whom the clinical evidence of intoxication is not clear-cut.

Decisions to screen for illicit substances should be taken by the multidisciplinary team in association with the patient and should be documented in a care plan. Arrangements for supervised collection, for example of urine samples, should give due consideration to the patient's dignity while minimising the opportunities for tampering with or substituting the sample. Test results should be interpreted with due caution in the light of advice from the relevant laboratory.

Non-coercive methods in the immediate management of violence

De-escalation and conflict management

Where aggression develops, de-escalation must represent a first intervention of a hierarchy of responses within the in-patient setting (Nyberg-Coles, 2005). The NHS Security Management Service (2005) in their best practice guidance, *Promoting Safer and Therapeutic Services*, defined a national syllabus for conflict resolution training for use in mental health. This syllabus forms the core of mandatory training for mental health service staff in managing violence delivered by NHS trusts across the country. A key learning outcome identified in this syllabus is that employees must be able to 'identify and demonstrate aspects of non-verbal de-escalation: verbal strategies and conflict resolution styles' (p. 11).

Stevenson (1991) defined de-escalation as a 'complex, interactive process in which a service user is redirected towards a calmer personal space' (p. 6). Becoming competent at de-escalation is in itself a sophisticated activity requiring much more than just a theoretical understanding of aggression. It cannot be considered in purely academic terms. The practitioner must undertake a developmental process, resulting in self-awareness and enabling the skills of de-escalation to become instinctive. Put simply, the practitioner must use their own personality and sense of self to actively engage the person in order to de-escalate the situation. Dix *et al* (2008) suggest three basic components for effective face-to-face de-escalation:

1   the assessment of the immediate situation
2   communication skills designed to facilitate cooperation
3   tactics aimed at problem-solving.

The NICE's 2005 guideline on the short-term management of disturbed/ violent behaviour gives a more detailed summary of the process and skills involved in successful verbal de-escalation.

Time-out

The practice of time-out is noted in the Royal College of Psychiatrists' 1995 report *Strategies for the Management of Disturbed and Violent Patients in*

Psychiatric Units, where it is viewed as a procedure 'whereby the patient is separated temporally from a rewarding environment as part of a planned and recorded therapeutic programme to modify behaviour' (p. 5). It is not detailed in the NICE 2005 guidelines.

We performed an up-to-date literature search using the same search criteria detailed by the team who produced the 2005 NICE guidelines as well as hand-searching of mental health journals. Most articles related to the use of time-out with children with behavioural problems. Only four new papers were found that commented on time-out in psychiatric populations and these were either observational or descriptive studies. None of these studies provided empirical evidence regarding the efficacy of the approach.

Chapter 15 of the Mental Health Act *Code of Practice* only notes that that there should be guidelines to distinguish between seclusion and psychological behaviour therapy interventions such as 'time-out' (Department of Health, 2008). However, in Chapter 18 of the previous code of practice, parameters for the use of time-out were detailed (Department of Health, 1999). It states that:

> 'time out is a behaviour modification technique which denies a patient, for a period of no more than 15 minutes, opportunities to participate in an activity or to obtain positive reinforcers immediately following an incident of unacceptable behaviour. The patient is then returned to his or her original environment. Time Out should never include the use of a locked room and should be clearly distinguished from seclusion which is for use in an emergency only and should never form part of a behavioural programme' (p. 88).

Specifically, time-out should:

- form part of a programme which enables the patient to achieve positive goals as well as reducing unwanted behaviour
- enable a patient, following a change of behaviour, to be subject to fewer restrictions
- ordinarily not take place in a room which is used for seclusion on other occasions
- be used only as part of a planned approach to managing a difficult or disturbed patient.

Observation

Observation is an intervention that is used both for the short-term management of disturbed/violent behaviour and to prevent self-harm. According to NICE, the primary aim of observation should be to engage positively with the patient. This involves 'a two-way relationship, established between a service user and a nurse, which is meaningful, grounded in trust, and therapeutic for the service user' (National Institute for Health and Clinical Excellence, 2005: p. 25). The recommendations and good practice points outlined below and adapted from NICE are specifically directed towards the use of observation as an intervention for the short-term management of disturbed/violent behaviour.

- The level of observation should be determined following a comprehensive assessment of risk. The observation level must be the least intrusive possible, commensurate with the level of risk identified.
- Four levels of observations are suggested by NICE. These are general, intermittent, within eyesight and within arms-length, and can be utilised in a step-wise manner when managing increasing levels of risk as assessed by early recognition of antecedents and warning signs.
- The observer must be competent and trained to undertake the task at hand and have sufficient knowledge of the patient, specific risks and the rationale behind the required level of observation. They must have the skills to engage with a patient in a positive manner as well as being able to recognise and manage disturbed behaviour.
- The level of observation should be reviewed on a regular basis and set out in local protocol, determining who within the team makes this decision and how frequently reviews take place.
- As far as possible, the patient should be involved in the decision-making process regarding the level of observation.
- Observing patients may be an intrusive exercise at times, so the clinical team needs to be sensitive to a patient's dignity and privacy while maintaining the safety of those around them.

Coercive interventions in the management of violence

Breakaway

Physical contact with violent patients is in some cases unavoidable and therefore training in breakaway techniques (physical skills to help separate or break away from an aggressor in a safe manner) can minimise harm and is recommended by NICE (2005). Despite training being mandatory in many mental healthcare settings for a number of years, the efficacy and transmissibility to clinical practice is not without controversy (Rogers *et al*, 2006; Dickens *et al*, 2009). In addition to local, mandatory, service-focused curriculums in breakaway training, the timing of training and frequency of refresher courses should be agreed by employers. It is known, for instance, that those new to working in mental healthcare settings and those working in more acute front-line settings are at higher risk of assault and so training should be directed towards these individuals. The content of training courses is also shifting towards a more readily retainable provision of fewer, adaptable techniques in an attempt to improve efficacy in practice (Dickens *et al*, 2009, 2012; Mott *et al*, 2009).

Evidence for and efficacy of methods of interpersonal restraint

The use of physical interventions, frequently referred to as restraint, is a widespread practice and often preferable to the use of seclusion. Organised approaches to the use of physical interventions have been developed with patient and staff safety in mind. The lack of consistency in the methods of restraint presents a major obstacle to an empirical evaluation of current practice and there is little evidence for its efficacy. However, much of the theoretical underpinning for the use of systemised restraint can be said to arise from common sense. Put simply, it must be preferable for staff to act in a consistent, coordinated fashion in relation to restraint than the alternative of an improvised spontaneous approach. The National Institute for Health and Care Excellence has reviewed much of the published evidence and its guidance (National Institute for Health and Clinical Excellence, 2005) is central to any consideration of how restraint should be practised and the major issues involved.

Safety

The very nature of aggression and restraint will always contain an element of unpredictability. It can reasonably be said that it may be impossible to account for all potential hazards in attempting to bring an often highly charged and frightening episode of physical aggression or disturbance under safe control. To maximise the safety of the person being restrained, a number of considerations have been proposed and it is helpful to consider these factors under two broad headings:

1   factors that are related to the person being restrained
2   factors that may emerge during the process of restraint.

Safety factors innate to the person being restrained

Wherever possible it is important that staff have a detailed knowledge of the person who may be subject to restraint. This is essential not only for minimising the need for physical intervention in the first place, but also to diminish the likelihood of injury or collapse. The following are important factors that need to be taken into account when considering the physical safety of a person being restrained:

- pre-existing medical conditions, especially cardiac or respiratory (e.g. heart disease, asthma)
- pre-existing skeletal or muscular injury or disease
- pregnancy
- extreme fear as a function of delusional beliefs
- obesity
- substance misuse
- high doses of medications.

In many circumstances it will be possible for staff to complete an assessment of the factors listed above before restraint is applied. This assessment should form part of multidisciplinary contingency planning in managing potential violence and should also involve the service user wherever possible.

Safety factors emerging during the process of restraint

Beyond the factors that the service user brings to the episode of restraint, the restraint process itself also requires close scrutiny to identify safety concerns that may emerge. It requires no great extension of common sense to recognise that even for an otherwise fit and healthy person, the spectacle of a violent struggle also poses serious risks. To manage these risks, constant awareness is required from staff involved in the restraint – often no easy task when their attention will inevitably be focused on bringing the situation under control.

There are a variety of important safety considerations which may emerge during the process of restraint that have been highlighted in evidence-based guidance (Parkes, 2002; Blofeld *et al*, 2003; Paterson & Leadbetter, 2004; Macpherson *et al*, 2005). The physical well-being of the restrained person should be a primary concern in the situations below.

- Prolonged restraint – the longer the restraint is applied, the greater the risk of serious harm or injury. Recommendation 9 of the inquiry into the death of David 'Rocky' Bennett in the Norvic Clinic in Norwich in 1998 stated that 'under no circumstances should any patient be restrained in a prone position for a longer period than three minutes' (Blofeld *et al*, 2003: p. 67). Mr Bennett died after being held face down on the floor for 28 min. National Institute for Health and Clinical Excellence guidelines chose not to specify a maximum time limit for physical restraint, because there was no conclusive evidence to suggest a specific maximum time limit for which patients could be safely restrained. Instead, NICE guidelines emphasised that the level of force used in managing violent patients must be justifiable, appropriate, reasonable and proportionate, and applied for the minimum possible amount of time.
- The prone position – body weight can directly restrict the mechanics of respiration when applied to either the front or back of the person being restrained.
- Increased body temperature – this can result from prolonged arousal and shared body heat between the restraining team and the service user.
- Inappropriate or poorly applied techniques – this can lead to an increased risk of injury, pain or serious harm.

Managing interpersonal restraint and the role of the medical emergency response team

Metherall *et al* (2006) described the creation of medical emergency response teams available to respond quickly to episodes of restraint over a 24-hour period. The medical emergency response team includes an assessor trained to intermediate life support standards, whose sole role is to monitor the physical condition of the service user being restrained.

In the event of prolonged restraint, a careful balance needs to be drawn between the risk to the service user of continuing restraint and the risk of further assault if restraint is discontinued. In some circumstances this may need to be weighted towards early discontinuation of restraint while accepting some risk of further assault. The role of the medical emergency response team assessor is to be aware of all the physical risk factors associated with restraint and to function as follows:

- to remain independent to the restraint team, with a priority in advocating for the service user's physical health
- to maintain communication with the staff member responsible for leading the restraint or holding the head of the service user during the restraint episode
- to monitor the airway, respiration and circulation of the service user, and whenever possible utilise pulse oximetry
- to ensure that the service user's well-being is monitored and physical observations are recorded and managed with awareness of peri-arrest criteria.

Although accepting the lack of quality evidence about the efficacy of restraint methods, there can be little excuse for not paying close attention to the known factors that have an impact on the safety of the service user during the restraint process. Provision for the close physical monitoring of the service user under restraint must be considered as a core principle underpinning best practice. Moreover, such provision is also recommended by NICE (2005). This philosophy can be easily extended to the safety of staff, which also needs a robust system of monitoring and audit, probably best described within existing health and safety and human resource procedures.

Leadership and restraint

Without skilled leadership in taking forward crisis resolution strategies, situations will often become much worse than they may have needed to be. Leadership is an essential part of avoiding the need for restraint through de-escalation and, when absolutely necessary, for its minimal and safe application. Unlike management, it is extremely difficult to set out a list of definitive measures that can be applied to produce effective clinical leaders, in particular in dealing with crises. The following are suggested as desirable characteristics:

- highly developed communication skills
- an ability to empathise with the service user and the wider staff team
- creative thinking towards options for resolving crises
- a willingness to take the initiative and to take the lead
- a calm and receptive attitude

- flexibility in overcoming potential conflict
- a willingness to take risks in allowing frustration discharge without quick resort to physical intervention
- the ability to facilitate service users and other staff in utilising crisis resolution skills.

Dignity

No matter how robust the justification, the experience of being physically restrained may be perceived by the service user as an assault on their dignity. In many cases where restraint is necessary, there will be an opportunity to take meaningful and practical steps towards promoting the dignity of the person. In some cases the need for restraint may arise spontaneously, leaving little time for planning. Often, however, there will be time to consider how best to minimise the distress that is likely to result. Simple steps include:

- careful consideration of the location for restraint
- minimising the likelihood that the process will be observed by onlookers
- the gender of the staff applying restraint should, where possible, be the same as the person being restrained.

In the case of giving rapid tranquillisation while under restraint, it will often be necessary to expose embarrassing parts of the body, in particular the upper outer quadrant of the buttock. The combination of being restrained while clothing is removed has the obvious potential to be perceived as sexual assault. Every effort should be made to ensure a gender match between staff and service user, particularly for female service users.

Seclusion

General principles

Seclusion is the supervised confinement of a patient in a room, which may be locked. Its sole aim is to contain severely disturbed behaviour which is likely to cause harm to others. Alternative phrases such as 'therapeutic isolation', 'single-person wards' and 'enforced segregation' should not be used so as to ensure that service users are protected by the safeguards built into the Mental Health Act *Code of Practice* (Department of Health, 2008). The code lists a number of requirements on managers and clinicians for the safe and appropriate use of seclusion. It should be used only as a last resort and for the shortest possible time. Seclusion should not be used as a punishment or a threat. A shortage of staff is in itself not a justification for the use of seclusion. In addition, it should not form part of a treatment programme, and post-incident support for patients and debriefing for staff is essential.

The use of seclusion compared with alternatives

Seclusion should always be considered a last resort when dealing with disturbed behaviour. About 50% of psychiatric intensive care units in the UK operate a no seclusion policy, as do many other wards in acute and secure settings. However, seclusion is still used in many UK in-patient services. As discussed earlier in this chapter, other methods of managing violence, both coercive and non-coercive, are available as an alternative to seclusion and may be preferable.

In line with the experience of many mental health workers, most, if not all, advocates of de-escalation accept that at best the technique can only dramatically reduce, rather than eradicate, physical violence. Some authors point out that verbal de-escalation is a complex process and during interaction the dynamics can easily work in the opposite direction, leading to an escalation of aggression. Evidence has shown that the use of seclusion can limit the progression of disruptive behaviour to actual violence. Although seclusion has been advocated as a quick and effective method of preventing progression towards physical assault, it must be accepted that a determined attempt at verbal de-escalation is an obvious first intervention, with the use of time-out if this fails.

The use of interpersonal restraint can reduce the need for seclusion. Staff can develop skills to hold a patient for a limited time until either verbal de-escalation or medication works. It appears that increased staffing levels are highly significant in reducing seclusion use. One explanation for this could be that if more staff are available, then restraint is more readily attempted than the use of seclusion. As highlighted earlier, prolonged restraint has been known to result in sudden death and many of the deaths that actually occur while a patient is in the seclusion room have been correlated with a violent struggle immediately before the patient was secluded. It may be reasonable to suggest that 40 min spent in a seclusion room may be preferable and safer for both the patient and staff when compared with the same length of time spent in physical restraint.

It is beyond question that rapid tranquillisation is largely effective in calming an agitated, angry and potentially assaultive patient. However, its use has been shown to produce distressing side-effects and is also correlated with sudden death. In high-risk cases, the use of seclusion may be deemed more appropriate that using tranquillisation with or without subsequent seclusion.

The extra care area

The use of an extra care area in which a single patient may receive intensive nursing intervention is advocated in the *Mental Health Policy Implementation Guide* (Department of Health, 2002) as an alternative to seclusion, and has become a popular method of managing acute disturbance. The principles of the extra care area appear to fulfil much of the function of seclusion by removing a patient, who is liable to assault others, from the general ward population. It also has the advantage of keeping staff in contact with the patient through the aggressive episode so that they can utilise de-escalation skills. The use of graded observation in the extra care area has been demonstrated to show that seclusion can be completely replaced.

The extra care area method is not without its problems when compared with seclusion. An unintended consequence is that patients receive positive reinforcement of their disturbed behaviour as a result of the special attention they receive from prolonged use of the extra care area. The extra care area can also be difficult for staffing in terms of the numbers needed and the danger of creating a ward within a ward.

Safe transport of high-risk patients between sites

Transfers from home to hospital, between hospitals or between hospital and court or prison are stressful and anxiety provoking for patients. There is a heightened risk of violence or absconding when a patient needs to be transferred against their will. A high level of cooperation between different groups of professionals is needed. The attendant potential for mistaken assumptions, miscommunication or misunderstanding may add to the patient's uncertainty. Such transitions therefore require careful risk assessment and management.

The Mental Health Act 1983 confers the authority of a constable on those with the responsibility of detaining and conveying a person under the Act. This means that they have the legal power to transport the patient against their will, using reasonable force if necessary, to prevent the threat of violence or escape. The Mental Health Act *Code of Practice* (chapter 11) provides guidance on conveying patients to hospital and between hospitals (Department of Health, 2008).

Escorting staff may have particular difficulty with high-risk patients who are being taken to court, high secure hospital or prison. A normal passenger vehicle lacks any barrier between the driver and passengers and has forward-facing seats, making restraint difficult to manage safely.

Transfers to a general hospital also pose problems:

- physical pain or discomfort may increase the patient's arousal
- there may be a prolonged wait for attention or investigations
- there are numerous exits
- potential weapons are easily available
- there are other vulnerable people in the vicinity.

Each high-risk patient should have a contingency plan detailing the measures to reduce the risk of absconding and of violence for such journeys. The patient should be involved in agreeing the contingency plan wherever possible. A planning meeting should take place beforehand. Simple measures such as restricting access to money and outdoor clothing should be considered as part of the risk management plan. Police assistance and advice should be sought where necessary. For long journeys the police may also assist by arranging for breaks en route in a secure police station.

The Prison Service may be able to provide an escort for high-risk patients on remand or for transfers to prison if given sufficient notice: if so, they will use Prison Service protocols in which the patient is handcuffed and attached to an officer (or, within hospital, to a stationary object) by security chain.

According to Department of Health best practice guidelines (Jobbins *et al*, 2007), medium secure services should have an approved policy for the safe transport of high-risk patients in addition to policies on escorts and Section 17 leave (specification for adult medium secure services).

Consideration should be given to using a secure vehicle and, if appropriate (e.g. in the case of high-risk transferred prisoners), physical restraints such as handcuffs.

Handcuffs

Handcuffs may increase as well as reduce risk (Box 4.1). They should only be used by hospital staff with appropriate training or by police or prison staff, and only if the risk is not manageable without them. Their use should never be routine. They cannot be used in cases of injury to the upper body or where unhampered access is needed for investigation or treatment of a physical condition.

Non-pharmacological management of violence in Black and minority ethnic patients

A disproportionate number of Black and minority ethnic (BME) patients have died as a result of excessive force, restraint or serious medical neglect. *Big, Black and Dangerous?* examined the deaths of Michael Martin, Joseph Watts and Orville Blackwood, who all died at Broadmoor Hospital after being placed in seclusion cells (Special Hospitals Services Authority, 1993). The report recognised many issues which affect all BME service users. The death of David 'Rocky' Bennett at the Norvic Clinic in October 1998 raised particular issues concerning the use of interpersonal restraint in BME patients. On the night of his death, Bennett was removed from his ward after fighting with another patient who had 'racially' abused him. While resisting the move, Bennett assaulted a nurse. Five nurses then used restraint measures, holding Bennett face down while immobilising his arms, ankles and upper chest for 28 min. After some time, the nurses realised that he was no longer struggling or breathing. They were not able to revive him and he was pronounced dead a short time later.

Bennett's death was described as just one example of racial discrimination and a 'festering abscess' within the NHS (Blofeld *et al*, 2003). The report noted, among other things, that the nurses were not

---

Box 4.1 Risks and benefits of using handcuffs during transport of high-risk patients

Risks

- Undermining therapeutic relationship with patient
- Stigmatising patient
- May facilitate assault (e.g. by strangling)
- Soft tissue injury to wrists
- Difficult to keep staff training current if rarely used
- May hamper treatment for physical condition

Benefits

- May prevent unplanned restraint in public
- May prevent rapid tranquillisation in unsafe surroundings (e.g. in vehicle)
- May prevent assault (by limiting reach and dexterity)
- May prevent absconding (by limiting ability to run or open doors)
- May be containing for the patient

---

aware of Bennett's cultural needs, that they treated him as a 'lesser being'. Research shows that BME people, particularly young African–Caribbean men, receive 'the harsher end' of mental healthcare, with more detention, more medication, more locked wards and less access to psychotherapy and counselling. There is also a history of misunderstanding, discrimination and bad practice in using coercive powers against African–Caribbean people (Mental Health Alliance, 2006). This in turn can be seen to propagate a 'circle of fear', driven by prejudicial treatment and a resultant mistrust of services by those in the BME population (Sainsbury Centre for Mental Health, 2002).

Likely causes for overuse of interpersonal restraint in BME patients

The following may be reasons for the more frequent use of coercive methods of management of violence:

- lack of cultural competence and sensitivity training among staff
- BME patients, particularly those who are African or African–Caribbean, may be perceived as 'dangerous', making the need to use force more likely
- preponderance of staff who are White found in some units; many do not attempt to understand the cultural needs of patients or fail to address identified relevant cultural issues
- BME patients may feel their needs are not being met
- a victim of racial abuse may feel acutely sensitive and have the desire to retaliate, particularly if their perception is that no action may be taken to prevent further racist abuse.

Measures to avoid adverse experiences in the BME population

We would suggest the following as simple practical steps which could be taken to better manage episodes of violence by BME patients. Many of these measures are not limited to the BME population and are suggested as good practice in managing all potentially violent episodes.

- There should be a time limit on physical restraint. The inquiry into the death of David Bennett recommended a maximum 3-minute time limit on prone restraint.
- All staff should be given adequate training in all forms of resuscitation techniques appropriate to their discipline and such training should be regularly updated.
- Promotion of an ethnically diverse workforce should be mandatory.
- Training of workforce in 'cultural competence and sensitivity' should be carried out by all services.
- Actions following aggression between a BME patient and other persons (whether from a BME group or not) should be such that justice can be seen to have been done. (David Bennett was further aggravated that no action was taken in respect of the other patient.)
- Concerns from BME patients should be acknowledged promptly by staff and advice should be sought from colleagues and senior members of staff when necessary.

Summary

- Engagement in structured, therapeutic activity rather than nursing in restricted, contained environments can prevent violence.
- Interpersonal relationships between staff and service users are invaluable in minimising aggression and aiding de-escalation.
- Risk assessment and planning can often allow for contingency planning prior to episodes of violence and, where possible, should involve the service user.
- When violence occurs, verbal de-escalation and management is often the safest, least harmful method of management.
- Time-out should be considered as a further non-coercive method.
- The level of nursing observation should reflect the level of risk faced and should aim to manage the situation without imposing on the service user's privacy.
- Coercive methods are in certain situations necessary to protect staff, other service users and the patient in question.
- The safe use of interpersonal restraint is of paramount importance. Medical emergency response team assessors should be present with the sole purpose of monitoring the physical condition of the service user.
- Seclusion may have a role in managing severely disturbed behaviour when other methods have failed.

- The cultural needs of BME patients should be taken into consideration when contingency planning and managing disturbed behaviour.

References

Abderhalden, C., Needham, I., Dassen, T., *et al* (2008) Structured risk assessment and violence in acute psychiatric wards: randomised controlled trial. *British Journal of Psychiatry*, **193**, 44–50.

Blofeld, J., Sallah, D., Sashidharan, S., *et al* (2003) *Independent Inquiry into the Death of David Bennett*. Cambridgeshire Strategic Health Authority.

Bowers, L., Simpson, A., Eyres, S., *et al* (2006) Serious untoward incidents and their aftermath in acute inpatient psychiatry: the Tompkins Acute Ward Study. *International Journal of Mental Health Nursing*, **15**, 226–234.

Cresswell, J. & Beavon, M. (eds) (2010) *Accreditation for Inpatient Mental Health Services (AIMS). Standards for Inpatient Wards – Working-age Adults* (4th edn). Royal College of Psychiatrists.

Department of Health (1999) *Code of Practice to the Mental Health Act 1983*. TSO (The Stationery Office).

Department of Health (2001) *The Mental Health Policy Implementation Guide*. Department of Health.

Department of Health (2002) *Mental Health Policy Implementation Guide: National Minimum Standards in Psychiatric Intensive Care Units (PICU) and Low Secure Environments*. Department of Health.

Department of Health (2008) *Code of Practice: Mental Health Act 1983*. TSO (The Stationery Office).

Dickens, G., Rogers, G., Rooney, C., *et al* (2009) An audit of the use of breakaway techniques in a large psychiatric hospital: a replication study. *Journal of Psychiatric and Mental Health Nursing*, **16**, 777–783.

Dickens, G., Rooney, C., Doyle, D., *et al* (2012) Breakaways in specialist secure psychiatry. *Journal of Psychiatric and Mental Health Nursing*, **19**, 281–284.

Dix, R., Betteridge, C. & Page, M. (2008) Seclusion: past, present and future. In *Psychiatric Intensive Care* (2nd edn) (eds D. Beer, S. M. Pereira & C. Paton), pp. 106–123. Cambridge University Press.

Janner, M. (2006) *Star Wards*. Old Rope Enterprises.

Jobbins, C., Abbott, B., Brammer, L., *et al* (2007) *Best Practice Guidance: Specification for Adult Medium-secure Services*. Department of Health.

Macpherson, R., Dix, R. & Morgan, S. (2005) A growing evidence base for management guidelines. Revisiting...Guidelines for the management of acutely disturbed psychiatric patients. *Advances in Psychiatric Treatment*, **11**, 404–415.

Mental Health Alliance (2006) *Briefing for the Second Reading of the Mental Health Bill in the House of Lords: Black and Minority Ethnic Mental Health Service Users*. MHA (http://www.mentalhealthalliance.org.uk/pre2007/documents/BME_Briefing_2nd_Reading.pdf).

Metherall, A., Worthington, R. & Keyte, A. (2006) Twenty four hour medical emergency response teams in a mental health in-patient facility – new approaches for safer restraint. *Journal of Psychiatric Intensive Care*, **2**, 21–29.

Mott, A., Dobson, P., Walton, J., *et al* (2009) Breakaway training for NHS staff: time for a fresh approach? *Journal of Mental Health Training, Education and Practice*, 4, 37–46.

National Institute for Health and Clinical Excellence (2005) *The Short-term Management of Disturbed/Violent Behaviour in In-patient Psychiatric Settings and Emergency Departments* (Clinical Guideline CG25). NICE.

NHS Security and Management Service (2005) *Promoting Safer and Therapeutic Services: Implementing the National Syllabus in Mental Health and Learning Disability Services*. NHS Security Management Service.

Nyberg-Coles, M. (2005) Promoting safer and therapeutic services. *Mental Health Practice*, **8**, 16–17.

Parkes, J. (2002) A review of the literature on positional asphyxia as a possible cause of sudden death during restraint. *British Journal of Forensic Practice*, **4**, 24–27.

Paterson, B. & Leadbetter, D. (2004) Learning the right lessons. *Mental Health Practice*, **7**, 12–15.

Rogers, P., Ghroum, P., Benson, R., *et al* (2006) Is breakaway training effective? An audit of one medium secure unit. *Journal of Forensic Psychiatry and Psychology*, **17**, 593–602.

Royal College of Psychiatrists (1995) *Strategies for the Management of Disturbed and Violent Patients in Psychiatric Units* (Council Report CR41). Royal College of Psychiatrists.

Sainsbury Centre for Mental Health (2002) *Breaking the Circles of Fear: A Review of the Relationship between Mental Health Services and African and Caribbean Communities*. SCMH.

Special Hospitals Services Authority (1993) *The Report of The Committee of Inquiry into the Death in Broadmoor Hospital of Orville Blackwood and a Review of the Deaths of Two Other Afro-Caribbean Patients: 'Big, Black and Dangerous?'*. SHSA.

Standing Nursing and Midwifery Advisory Committee (1999) *Mental Health Nursing: Addressing Acute Concerns*. Department of Health.

Stevenson, S. (1991) Heading off violence with verbal de-escalation. *Journal of Psychosocial Nursing & Mental Health Services*, **29**, 6–10.

van de Sande, R., Nijman, H. L. I., Noorthoorn, E. O., *et al* (2011) Aggression and seclusion on acute psychiatric wards: effect of short-term risk assessment. *British Journal of Psychiatry*, **199**, 473–478.

CHAPTER 5

Use of medication and ECT in the management of violence

Caroline Parker, Masum Khwaja and Jonathan Waite

Our guidance will focus on the use of medication as an emergency response – i.e. rapid tranquillisation – but we will also briefly discuss the use of medication in the management of the risk of violence in the medium to longer term. We suggest that our guidance is read in conjunction with the 2005 NICE guidelines.

General principles for prescribing medication to prevent or control violence

The use of medication in the control of violence is only one part of a comprehensive treatment plan to manage the risk of violence that includes an assessment of environmental factors and the use of other therapies.

Medication should not be used to manage aggression caused by identifiable environmental factors (such as understaffing or lack of staff skills) that can be dealt with by other means.

Good practice principles in prescribing medication to prevent or control violence include the list below.

- Medication should only be used when the risk of not using medication is judged to be greater than that arising from its use.
- The indication for which any *pro re nata* (p.r.n.) medication is prescribed should be clearly stated.
- The lowest dose compatible with effective treatment should be used.
- The dose prescribed should be individually tailored for each patient; for example, older patients generally require lower doses of antipsychotic medication, and comorbid physical disorders and concomitant medication may influence the dose (and type) of medication prescribed.
- The choice of medication used should also be individually tailored to the patient and informed by a knowledge of their psychiatric and medical history, mental and physical state, treatment history, any existing advanced directive, and after an attempt has been made to establish a provisional diagnosis.

- As few medicines as possible should be used.
- The use of combinations from the same class of medicine is often unnecessary and should be avoided if possible.
- Patients should be regularly monitored for side-effects of medication, and both regular and as required (p.r.n.) medication should be reviewed on a regular basis.
- If there is evidence that the medicines prescribed are unnecessary or ineffective then they should be reduced and discontinued.
- The use of medicines outside their licence, or above maximum recommended dosage (either alone or in combination), is the responsibility of the individual practitioner who should undertake the recommended safeguards in relation to documentation of indications and consent.

The use of medicines outside their licence or above maximum recommended dosage (either alone or in combination)

A consensus statement on the use of high-dose antipsychotics in the longer-term management of schizophrenia was produced by the Royal College of Psychiatrists in 2006. Although the statement did not specifically address the emergency use of antipsychotics for rapid tranquillisation, the opinion expressed that the use of above *British National Formulary* (BNF) maximum doses of medication for treatment, whether in the context of violence or otherwise, should be carefully evaluated and justified, remains valid when considering prescribing medication to prevent or control violence. High doses of medication are unlikely to be routinely indicated for rapid tranquillisation. Furthermore, the appropriate use of benzodiazepines and possibly promethazine is likely to reduce the need to use above BNF maximum doses of antipsychotic.

The NICE guidelines (2005) on the short-term management of disturbed/violent behaviour in psychiatric in-patient settings and emergency departments state (p. 15):

'It is recognised that clinicians may decide that the use of medication outside of the Summary of Product Characteristics (SPC) is occasionally justified, bearing in mind the overall risks. However where the regulatory authorities or manufacturer issues a specific warning that this may result in an increased risk of fatality, the medication should only be used strictly in accordance with the current marketing authorisation.

In certain circumstances, current British National Formulary (BNF) uses and limits and the manufacturer's SPC may be knowingly exceeded (for example, for lorazepam). This decision should not be taken lightly or the risks underestimated. Record a risk–benefit analysis in the case notes and a rationale in the care plan. Where the risk–benefit is unclear, advice may be sought from clinicians not directly involved in the service user's care.

If current BNF doses or SPC are exceeded: it is particularly important to undertake frequent and intensive monitoring of a calmed service user, pay particular attention to regular checks of airway, level of consciousness, pulse, blood pressure, respiratory effort, temperature and hydration.'

Use of medication to reduce
the medium- and long-term risk of violence

There are two major obstacles in using the evidence available to support the prescribing of medication to specifically control the medium- and longer-term risk of violence, as opposed to treating symptoms of the primary disorder that might be related to a risk of violence.

First, the aetiology of violence is complex and a number of social and environmental factors might cause violence independently of the psychopathology of the patient (Swanson *et al*, 2008). For example, in individuals with psychotic disorders and symptoms, where the risk of violence is elevated, the risk may be unrelated to psychotic symptoms such as delusions (Applebaum *et al*, 2000) and may be related to prospective predictors of violence such as childhood conduct problems, substance misuse, victimisation history, economic deprivation and social living situation (Swanson *et al*, 2008).

Second, the evidence base for prescribing medication specifically to reduce violence in the medium- to longer-term is limited (Goedhard *et al*, 2006). There is clinical evidence that clozapine reduces aggression in schizophrenia and schizoaffective disorder (Chengappa, 2002; Volavka *et al*, 2004; Krakowski *et al*, 2006), and that the reduction in hostility and aggression may be independent of its antipsychotic effect (Kraus & Sheitman, 2005; Krakowski *et al*, 2006). Clozapine has also been shown to markedly reduce aggressive behaviour in in-patients with schizophrenia over 12 weeks (Krakowski *et al*, 2008). A second 12-week study indicated that clozapine was superior to olanzapine, and olanzapine was superior to haloperidol in reducing aggression (Krakowski & Czobor, 2011).

There is also some evidence that mood stabilisers and in particular carbamazepine might be a useful adjunctive treatment for assaultive patients with schizophrenia (Brieden *et al*, 2002). However, the evidence is insufficient to make any clear recommendations.

Compared with the relationship between schizophrenia and violence, the relationship between mood disorders and violence has been comparatively overlooked (Oakley *et al*, 2009). The relationship is likely to be as complex as with schizophrenia, and other than prescribing for the primary disorder, no specific recommendations are made.

With regard to personality disorders, NICE guidelines for borderline personality disorder (2009*a*) recommend: 'drug treatment should not be used specifically for borderline personality disorder or for the individual symptoms or behaviour associated with the disorder' (p. 10). Similarly, NICE guidelines for the management of antisocial personality disorder (2009*b*) recommend: 'pharmacological interventions should not be routinely used for the treatment of antisocial personality disorder or associated behaviours of aggression, anger and impulsivity' (p. 28). However, in practice medication is often prescribed in the treatment of personality disorder to treat comorbid disorders or to target particularly worrying symptoms that may increase the risk of aggression, especially in those with high levels of arousal that cannot be reduced by environmental, behavioural or other therapeutic methods. If medication is to be prescribed, a sensible approach is to consider a targeted symptom-specific prescribing (Soloff, 1998; Tyrer & Bateman, 2004).

Medication is also widely used in the management of patients with aggression after a head injury. The choice of medication to reduce aggression is often guided by the underlying hypothesised mechanism of action or by associated symptoms and the use of medicines should be considered in two categories: the treatment of the underlying disorder (e.g. depression) and the treatment of aggression. A partial response should lead to consideration of adjunctive treatment with a medicine that has a different mechanism of action (Jacobson, 1997).

Medication is increasingly used in the treatment of sexual deviancy disorders. The relationship of any coexisting mental disorder that may influence the risk of sexual offending may establish a need for pharmacological treatment and the potential for violence is one of several factors taken into consideration when deciding whether to prescribe or not. Psychotropic medication such as selective serotonin reuptake inhibitor antidepressants and hormonal medicines such as cyproterone acetate are increasingly used in men to diminish deviant sexual fantasies, urges and behaviours, and to reduce the risk of further victimisation (Gordon & Grubin, 2004). If medication is prescribed other than to treat a coexisting mental disorder that would normally require pharmacological treatment, it should be in addition to psychological treatment and then in general only when other non-pharmacological treatments used alone have proved insufficient. If treatment involves hormonal implants, then it should be given only in accordance with Section 57 of the Mental Health Act 1983.

Medication is used in the management of challenging behaviour in people with dementia. Of the different symptoms that constitute behavioural and psychological symptoms in dementia, only physical aggression has been shown to respond to medication (Ballard *et al*, 2006). The NICE guidelines (National Collaborating Centre for Mental Health, 2007) state that once certain conditions have been met, 'people with Alzheimer's disease, vascular dementia, mixed dementias or [dementia with Lewy bodies] with severe non-cognitive symptoms (psychosis and/or agitated behaviour causing significant distress) may be offered treatment with an antipsychotic drug' (p. 35). Risperidone is the only antipsychotic licensed for the treatment of aggression in people with dementia.

In summary, in prescribing medication to specifically target the medium- or long-term risk of violence, as opposed to symptoms of the patient's primary disorder that may be related to violence, the clinician should bear in mind the limited evidence base and the multifactorial aetiology of violent behaviour, and only prescribe medication following a careful multidisciplinary assessment and risk–benefit evaluation.

Use of ECT to control violence

Electroconvulsive therapy (ECT) is not a practicable or a desirable measure to treat violence or the risk of violence in an emergency situation.

The use of ECT in clinical practice is now guided by the Royal College of Psychiatrists' *The ECT Handbook* (Waite & Easton, 2013) and NICE guidelines (2003, 2009c). The NICE guidelines recommend that ECT should be used for acute treatment of severe depression that is life-threatening and when a rapid response is required, or when other treatments have failed; for people with moderate depression whose depression has not responded to multiple drug treatments and psychological treatment; or for prolonged or severe episodes of mania or catatonia.

Although NICE does not recommend the use of ECT in the general management of schizophrenia, ECT remains an option rarely used for some patients with treatment-resistant schizophrenia when other treatments have failed or there is a known history of good response to ECT (Tharyan & Adams, 2005). Furthermore, *The ECT Handbook* recommends that ECT may be considered as a fourth-line option – that is, for patients with schizophrenia for whom clozapine has already proven ineffective or intolerable.

Once an indication for ECT has been established, the potential for violence should be one of a range of factors to consider in terms of the risks *v*. benefits of giving ECT.

Valid consent for ECT must be obtained in all cases where the patient has capacity to do so. The decision to use ECT should be made jointly by the patient and the responsible clinician on the basis of an informed discussion. This discussion should be enabled by the provision of full and appropriate information about the general risks associated with ECT and about the risks and potential benefits specific to that patient. Consent should be obtained without pressure or coercion, which may occur as a result of the circumstances and clinical setting, and the patient should be reminded of their right to withdraw consent at any point. There should be strict adherence to recognised guidelines about consent and the involvement of patient advocates and/or carers to facilitate informed discussion is strongly encouraged. In all situations where informed discussion and consent is not possible, advance directives should be taken fully into account and the patient's advocate and/or carer consulted.

Section 58A of the Mental Health Act applies to ECT and to medication administered as part of ECT. It applies to detained patients and to all patients aged under 18 (whether or not detained). A patient who has capacity to consent may not be given ECT under Section 58A unless the approved clinician in charge, or a SOAD appointed by the Care Quality Commission, has certified that the patient has the capacity to consent and has done so. If the patient is under 18, only a SOAD may give the certificate, and the SOAD must certify that the treatment is appropriate.

A patient who lacks capacity to consent may not be given treatment under Section 58A unless a SOAD certifies that the patient lacks capacity to consent and that: treatment is appropriate; no valid and applicable advance decision has been made by the patient under the Mental Capacity Act 2005 refusing the treatment; no suitably authorised attorney or deputy objects to the treatment on the patient's behalf; and as long as the treatment would not conflict with a decision of the Court of Protection. The Care Quality Commission expects the clinical team making the referral to have checked that there is no conflict with a proxy decision maker or any advance decision to refuse treatment, as a condition of the SOAD visit (Care Quality Commission, 2008).

In emergency situations, ECT may be given for two of the four situations mentioned in Section 62 of the Mental Health Act: treatment, which (not being irreversible or hazardous) is immediately necessary to alleviate serious suffering by the patient; or, which (not being irreversible or hazardous) is immediately necessary and represents the minimum interference necessary to prevent the patient from behaving violently or being a danger to himself or to others.

Rapid tranquillisation

As defined in the NICE guideline on violence and aggression (2005: p. 100), rapid tranquillisation is:

> 'All medication given in the short-term management of disturbed/violent behaviour should be considered as part of rapid tranquillisation (including [PRN] medication).'

Principles of prescribing medicines in rapid tranquillisation

The aim of rapid tranquillisation is to quickly calm the severely agitated patient in order to reduce the risk of imminent and serious violence to self or others. Rapid tranquillisation is not trying to treat the underlying psychiatric condition.

Following rapid tranquillisation the patient should be calm and still able to participate in further assessment and treatment. The aim of rapid tranquillisation is not to induce sleep or unconsciousness, although there may be occasions when sedation is an appropriate goal. The patient should be able to respond to communication throughout.

Any medication used by a team caring for a patient who requires rapid tranquillisation needs to be carefully considered to ensure that it is capable of achieving these aims with the minimum distress and risk to the patient and staff.

Environmental and situational factors can influence behaviour and need to be considered and addressed (e.g. through de-escalation techniques; National Institute for Health and Clinical Excellence, 2005).

Consideration should also be given to any coexisting medical illnesses and conditions, as some may predispose the patient to agitated or dysphoric states, for example severe constipation in the elderly, urinary tract infections which may lead to confusion, akathisia, unmanaged pain, and other dysphoric states. In such circumstances the underlying state should be treated accordingly.

Prior to prescribing rapid tranquillisation, consideration should also be given to any coexisting regularly prescribed medication (oral/depot), and the recent use of any illicit substances, as prescribed or illicit drugs may interact either pharmacodynamically or pharmacokinetically with the proposed rapid-tranquillisation medications, leading to altered dose requirements and potential side-effects.

Where there is documentation in the patient's care plan of their preference in medication to be used in the event of an acute episode of illness (an advance directive), this preference should be adhered to if clinically appropriate. The care programme approach coordinator should ensure that the individual's advance directive is notified to the prescribers during the acute phase of illness. In all cases the patient must be informed that medication is going to be given and must be provided the opportunity at any stage to accept oral medication voluntarily. All patients should be given the opportunity to make an informed choice where at all possible.

For all patients, wherever practicable, consent to medical treatment should always be sought and consent or refusal recorded. The capacity to give consent should also be assessed and documented clearly in the patient's notes. If the patient has given consent and has capacity to do so, then treatment can of course be given.

The Mental Capacity Act, the common law doctrine of necessity and an evaluation of 'best interests' are all relevant when considering the legality of administering rapid tranquillisation to a patient who is refusing treatment or lacks capacity to consent to treatment. Sections 5 and 6 of the Mental Capacity Act provide a defence against liability in relation to acts such as restraining mentally incapacitated adults using reasonable force or giving them medication without consent, which is necessary in their best interests. Where treatment or restraint is necessary not because it is in the patient's best interests but for the protection of others, defence would come from the common law doctrine of necessity.

The procedure for determining the best interests of a person with impaired capacity is laid down in Section 4 of the Mental Capacity Act. This takes into account any valid advanced decisions and statements, the patient's past and present feelings, beliefs and values likely to influence their decision, and any other factors which they would be likely to consider if able to do so. If practicable and appropriate, the views of anyone named by the patient, such as a carer or person interested in their welfare, must also be consulted.

For detained patients for whom Part IV of the Mental Health Act applies, Section 63 permits medication for mental disorder to be given to patients detained under certain sections of the Act (e.g. Sections 2, 3, 36, 37, 37/41, 38, 45A, 47 or 48), but only if the patient has given valid consent and has capacity to do so or, if the patient is incapable and/or refusing, medication is given by or under the direction of the approved clinician in charge of the treatment in question. Medication can then be given for up to 3 months from the date medication was first administered. Section 58 applies to the administration of medication for mental disorder once 3 months have passed from the date it was first administered to a detained patient, the so-called 'three-month rule'. This includes any time the patient has spent on SCT. Medication can then only be given if the patient consents, treatment is approved by a SOAD or in an emergency situation under Section 62:

- treatment which is immediately necessary to save the patient's life
- treatment (not being irreversible or hazardous) which is immediately necessary to prevent a serious deterioration in their condition
- treatment (not being irreversible or hazardous) which is immediately necessary to alleviate serious suffering by the patient
- treatment (not being irreversible or hazardous) which is immediately necessary and represents the minimum interference necessary to prevent the patient from behaving violently or being a danger to himself or to others.

Detained persons not covered by Part IV of the Mental Health Act include:

- those detained on 'emergency' sections of the Act (e.g. Sections 4, 5, 135 and 136)
- those remanded to hospital for a report under Section 35, patients temporarily detained in hospital as a place of safety under Section 37 or 45A pending admission to the hospital named in their hospital order or hospital direction
- restricted patients who have been conditionally discharged (unless or until recalled).

These patients are in the same position as patients who are not subject to the Mental Health Act at all. They have the same rights consenting to treatment as if they were not detained and therefore treatment can only be given, as described earlier, following an assessment of capacity, an evaluation of best interests, and the principles enshrined in the Mental Capacity Act and the common law doctrine of necessity.

Patients on supervised community treatment

If treatment is required as part of the management of violent behaviour, it is likely that the emergency provisions of the Mental Health Act (Sections 62A and 64G) will apply.

Patients with capacity

For patients with capacity, the responsible clinician must complete Form CTO12 within 1 month of the CTO start date to certify that the patient both has capacity to consent to treatment and does consent to treatment (Mental Health Act Section 64C). There is no authority under the Act to give medication to a capacitous patient on SCT against their will in the community, even in an emergency. Treatment without their consent can only legally be given if they are recalled to hospital.

Patients lacking capacity

All treatment given in the community to a patient on SCT lacking capacity (except in an emergency) after the first month must be certified by a SOAD and documented on Form CTO11.

Patients on SCT who lack capacity to consent to treatment may be given medication without their consent in the community, provided they have not made an advance decision by which they refuse such treatment (Mental Capacity Act Section 24), and no proxy decision maker such as a deputy appointed by the court (Mental Capacity Act Sections 16–20) or holder of a lasting power of attorney (Mental Capacity Act Sections 9–11) objects. Treatment may also be given in the above circumstances if the patent does object, but force is not required in order to give the treatment (Mental Health Act Section 64D).

In an emergency, Section 64G of the Mental Health Act permits the administration of medicine which is immediately necessary to:

- save the patient's life
- prevent serious deterioration
- alleviate serious suffering by the patient
- prevent the patient behaving violently or being a danger to themselves or others, where the treatment represents the minimum interference necessary for that purpose, does not have unfavourable psychological consequences which cannot be reversed and does not entail significant physical hazard.

There is no requirement for the person giving treatment to be acting under the direction of an approved clinician – force may be used provided that:

- the treatment is necessary to prevent harm to the patient
- the force used is proportionate to the likelihood of the patient suffering harm and to the seriousness of that harm.

Treatment under Section 64G might be considered where the possibility of recall to hospital before commencing treatment is not realistic or might exacerbate the patient's condition.

Treatment of patients on SCT after recall to hospital

Such patients are 'detained patients' within the meaning of Part IV of the Mental Health Act. Their treatment is governed by Section 62A.

There are three circumstances in which medication may legally be given to recalled patients on SCT.

1   If the treatment has been specifically allowed on recall by the SOAD and documented on the Part IVA certificate (Section 62A(3)(a)).
2   If less than 1 month has elapsed since the CTO was made (Section 62A(3)(b)).
3   If the treatment was already being given on the authority of a Part IVA certificate and the person in charge of treatment believes that stopping the treatment would cause serious suffering (Section 62A(3)(b)).

Treatment may be continued in these circumstances while awaiting approval from a SOAD for a new treatment plan.

In the absence of such circumstances, Part IV of the Mental Health Act resumes and Section 62 is applicable.

Route of administration of medicines in rapid tranquillisation

In general, oral medication should be offered before parenteral treatment is administered, although parenterally administered medication has a faster onset of action.

A number of the newer atypical antipsychotics are available as soluble or disintegrating tablets (aripiprazole, risperidone and olanzapine) as well as liquids (amisulpride, aripiprazole and risperidone). However, it should be noted that the medication is not buccally absorbed from these formulations; the tablets disperse in the saliva and on swallowing are absorbed via the gastrointestinal tract.

It is strongly recommended that oral and intramuscular medicines should be prescribed separately on prescription charts, and the abbreviation 'p.o./i.m.' (oral/intramuscular) should not be used, as parenteral and oral doses of a medication may not be bioequivalent and have different onsets of action. Oral and parenteral haloperidol and procyclidine are not bioequivalent.

If oral medication is repetitively refused, the decision to forcibly medicate a patient should be made jointly by medical and nursing staff directly involved with the patient's care. The decision to forcibly medicate should include a discussion as to whether medication can be legally enforced.

Once the decision has been made to forcibly medicate, the patient must be isolated from other patients on the ward and nursed in a side room. Nursing and medical staff involved in physically restraining the patient should be proficient in 'control and restraint' techniques, should have adequate immunisation against hepatitis B, and should ensure adequate physical restraint before attempting parenteral administration in a struggling patient.

Following the administration of parenteral medication, further doses of medicines should be given orally at the earliest opportunity.

In view of the safety considerations and the actual practical considerations of restraint and administration of boluses, intravenous rapid tranquillisation is not recommended in 'stand-alone' or isolated psychiatric settings, especially when there is no provision to call an experienced medical resuscitation team.

Intravenous haloperidol is associated with cardiac conduction abnormalities such as Torsade de pointes (Hassaballa & Balk, 2003*a,b*), and in general the use of intravenous and high doses of antipsychotics is of concern because of the potential to increase QT interval and the associated risk of tachyarrhythmias, which are likely to be contributing factors to unexplained sudden deaths of acutely disturbed patients prescribed antipsychotics.

The use of benzodiazepines carries a risk of respiratory depression, and with intravenous diazepam there is a high risk of thrombophlebitis (reduced by using an emulsion formulation).

Furthermore, in routine practice, if parenteral administration is required there are few situations where intramuscular injections are inappropriate. It is harder to administer an intravenous injection to a struggling and restrained patient as the injection site is specific and there is a risk of inadvertent intra-arterial administration, whereas an intramuscular injection does not require such a small injection site. The onset of action following an intramuscular injection is approximately 15 min, whereas onset of action following an intravenous injection is approximately 2–5 min. Parenteral intravenous rapid tranquillisation medications such as diazepam or haloperidol, as opposed to intramuscular, need to be given as slow boluses over at least 2–3 min. In addition, NICE guidelines on violence (National Institute for Health and Clinical Excellence, 2005) recommend that intravenous rapid tranquillisation should only occur with easy access to the full support resuscitation equipment. Furthermore, registered mental health nurses cannot administer intravenous doses unless they have completed additional training, meaning that any intravenous doses need to be administered by a doctor. Last, staff in many psychiatric units are unlikely to have the experience required to administer medicines safely by this route or manage the potentially serious side-effects of intravenous rapid tranquillisation should they arise.

Choice of agent in rapid tranquillisation

Although there are numerous reviews and commentaries on the subject (Battaglia, 2005; Aupperle, 2006; Caine, 2006; Marder, 2006; Parker & Khwaja, 2011), due to the acute nature of the clinical situation and the degree of risk of violence from the patient to themselves and others, it is notable that there are very few rigorous trials examining or comparing the efficacy and safety of agents in rapid tranquillisation, with a few exceptions (Gillies *et al*, 2010) such as the TREC trials (TREC Collaborative Group, 2003; Alexander *et al*, 2004; Huf *et al*, 2007; Raveendran *et al*, 2007). Therefore much of the data that informs practice are derived from naturalistic studies and case series; many published recommendations are consensuses of opinions (Allen *et al*, 2005) based on experience in clinical practice (Taylor *et al*, 2009).

Studies suggest that using a benzodiazepine alone is at least as effective as using an antipsychotic alone; additionally, using a benzodiazepine

45

alone is just as effective as using it in combination with an antipsychotic (Gillies *et al*, 2010; Isbister *et al*, 2010). However, other studies suggest to the contrary, and in more severe cases it is common practice to use a benzodiazepine (usually lorazepam) in conjunction with an antipsychotic (usually haloperidol). Two studies (Huf *et al*, 2007; Raveendran *et al*, 2007) suggest that the combination of haloperidol and promethazine is more effective than using antipsychotics alone. Furthermore, the addition of a benzodiazepine or promethazine to an antipsychotic gives rise to fewer adverse effects than using an antipsychotic alone, and requires the use of less additional medication (Huf *et al*, 2007; Gillies *et al*, 2010). These data shape the recommendations below.

- In general, a short-acting benzodiazepine is recommended as the first-line pharmacological treatment in rapid tranquillisation, whether orally or parenterally (Goedhard *et al*, 2006; Gillies *et al*, 2010). This has been shown to have equal efficacy to other options, and lower incidence of extrapyramidal side-effects (EPS). If this alone is insufficient, it may be appropriate to add an antipsychotic.
- As there is little difference in efficacy (Gillies *et al*, 2010) between benzodiazepines and antipsychotics, and considering the risk of EPS, cardiac arrhythmia and potential cardiorespiratory collapse, and the potentially life-threatening and unpredictable risk of neuroleptic malignant syndrome, antipsychotics are not recommended as first-line or sole agents in rapid tranquillisation (Huf *et al*, 2011). It is recommended that antipsychotics should be used in conjunction with benzodiazepines such as lorazepam, in order to increase the sedation as well as minimise the dose of antipsychotic required, and therefore the level of EPS experienced with typical antipsychotics. The combination of an antipsychotic with a benzodiazepine is more effective than using either agent alone.
- Although the aim of rapid tranquillisation is to manage the immediate acute situation and not treat the underlying condition, the provisional diagnosis may guide the choice of medication in rapid tranquillisation. For example, if there is diagnostic uncertainty, a clinician may prefer to avoid antipsychotic medication if possible, until the diagnosis is established. Another example would be if the patient has a diagnosis of schizophrenia, as then the clinician may decide to use an antipsychotic in preference to an anxiolytic, as they may consider it likely that post rapid tranquillisation antipsychotic medication will be prescribed on a regular basis.
- Knowledge of previous exposure to medications for rapid tranquillisation may also guide the choice of medication used. For example, if there is evidence that the patient has previously demonstrated a good response to oral clonazepam, then this may be the preferred option. Conversely, if the patient has previously shown disinhibited behaviour in response to a benzodiazepine, then an antipsychotic alone may be preferred.

- If benzodiazepines are contraindicated, for example in patients who have significant respiratory impairment or benzodiazepine tolerance, and yet pharmacological rapid tranquillisation is warranted, then an antipsychotic alone is recommended (oral or intramuscular) (Isbister *et al*, 2010).
- Antipsychotics more likely to cause EPS such as haloperidol should be avoided where possible in patients previously untreated with antipsychotics (antipsychotic-naive patients) and those with an unknown treatment history, due to the high incidence of EPS. If they are used, this should be done with caution and an oral and parenteral antimuscarinic should be made available to reduce the risk of EPS.
- NICE guidelines (2005) state that when using intramuscular haloperidol as a means of managing disturbed/violent behaviour, an antimuscarinic agent such as procyclidine or benzatropine should be immediately available to reduce the risk of dystonia and other EPS, as per the manufacturer's recommendations.
- In general, if a patient is accepting oral medication, this should be offered. Only parenteral options currently available for routine UK practice will be discussed in more detail.

Intramuscular antipsychotics

Haloperidol
Since the withdrawal of droperidol injection from the UK market in 2001 (Current Problems in Pharmacovigilance, 2001) following the meta-analysis by Reilly *et al* (2000), haloperidol is now recognised as the mainstay parenteral antipsychotic in rapid tranquillisation in the UK (Allen *et al*, 2005; National Institute for Health and Clinical Excellence, 2005) and is probably the most studied (TREC Collaborative Group, 2003; Alexander *et al*, 2004; Huf *et al*, 2007; Raveendran *et al*, 2007). It has a relatively fast onset of action, but EPS remain problematic.

Olanzapine
Intramuscular olanzapine has similar efficacy to intramuscular haloperidol when used as a single agent for acute agitation (Hsu *et al*, 2010; Baldacara *et al*, 2011), but the incidence of EPS is much lower with olanzapine than haloperidol (Belgamwar & Fenton, 2005), making it a preferable intramuscular antipsychotic for use in patients with a history of EPS. However, its main drawback is that simultaneous administration with parenteral benzodiazepines is unlicensed (Eli Lilly, 2009), owing to concern about patient safety. The safety of this practice was not formally assessed prior to licensing (Wright *et al*, 2001), and post-licensing a number of patient deaths occurred where intramuscular olanzapine was used in conjunction with several other agents, including benzodiazepines (Eli Lilly, 2004). In trials, single doses commonly (1–10%) caused postural hypotension, bradycardia with or without hypotension or syncope, and tachycardia,

and more uncommonly (0.1–1%), sinus pause and hypoventilation (Eli Lilly, 2009). If a patient additionally requires a parenteral benzodiazepine, this should not be given until at least 1h after intramuscular olanzapine (Eli Lilly, 2009) or *vice versa*, which raises significant issues in terms of clinical practice. The combination of olanzapine with promethazine has not been formally reported, and the use of intramuscular olanzapine alone is not as effective as the combination of intramuscular haloperidol and intramuscular promethazine (Raveendran *et al*, 2007).

Aripiprazole

This was licensed in the UK in 2007 with initial minimal uptake and therefore UK clinical experience is still low. Like olanzapine, this injectable atypical antipsychotic has shown in trials to have similar efficacy yet a significantly lower incidence of EPS than seen with haloperidol (Andrezina *et al*, 2006; Tran-Johnson *et al*, 2007; Zimbroff *et al*, 2007). However, unlike olanzapine it has been shown to be safe to give concurrently with parenteral benzodiazepines which are generally recommended as first-line treatment in rapid tranquillisation, therefore it is anticipated that aripiprazole injection potentially has a greater place in therapy than olanzapine.

Other licensed intramuscular agents in the UK

Lorazepam

This is the most widely used benzodiazepine for rapid tranquillisation in the UK and is frequently used in rapid tranquillisation studies. It is available as a tablet that may be taken orally or sublingually, as well as an injection for intramuscular administration. It is readily and completely absorbed from the gastrointestinal tract after oral administration, reaches peak plasma levels at approximately 2 h, and is quickly absorbed after intramuscular injection (unlike diazepam). It is one of the short-acting benzodiazepines, it does not have any active metabolites and its hepatic metabolism is not significantly impaired by hepatic dysfunction. Like all benzodiazepines, lorazepam may cause respiratory depression (Broadstock, 2001).

In some countries the practical requirement to store lorazepam injection in refrigerated conditions (2–8°C) to maintain stability of the product can prove to be inhibitory in medical settings.

Promethazine

Promethazine is a sedating antihistamine. It has been studied alongside intramuscular haloperidol as an alternative agent to a parenteral benzodiazepine such as lorazepam (Huf *et al*, 2007). The four large TREC trials (TREC Collaborative Group, 2003; Alexander *et al*, 2004; Huf *et al*, 2007; Raveendran *et al*, 2007) methodically demonstrated the relative safety and efficacy of the promethazine–haloperidol combination *v*. intramuscular midazolam, *v*. intramuscular lorazepam, *v*. intramuscular haloperidol alone, and *v*. intramuscular olanzapine, in a range of settings.

In this combination, promethazine showed benefits as a sedative (the promethazine–haloperidol combination was more sedating that using haloperidol alone), with a relatively swift onset of action and potentially a protective effect against haloperidol-induced EPS (Huf *et al*, 2007). A Cochrane review of the four TREC trials concluded that this was a useful agent in rapid tranquillisation (Huf *et al*, 2011).

Promethazine injection is licensed in the UK for intramuscular administration and for 'sedation', therefore from a medico-legal perspective it would be preferable to use this licensed option rather than administer intramuscular midazolam injection in an unlicensed manner.

Other unlicensed agents in the UK

Midazolam: intramuscular

The benzodiazepine midazolam is a schedule 3 controlled drug and it is licensed and commonly used in the UK as an intravenous sedative and induction anaesthetic. Intramuscular use of midazolam has also been investigated for rapid tranquillisation. This is widely used in some countries where the requirement to store lorazepam injection in refrigerated conditions inhibits the use of lorazepam.

In some studies, midazolam has shown to have a faster onset of action than lorazepam (Nobay *et al*, 2004; Huf *et al*, 2007) and some antipsychotics (Nobay *et al*, 2004; Martel *et al*, 2005) and has a shorter duration of action (Nobay *et al*, 2004). It can unpredictably lead to respiratory depression more frequently than other agents (TREC Collaborative Group, 2003; Martel *et al*, 2005; Isbister *et al*, 2010) and therefore it should only be used in scenarios where services are fully confident in observing for and managing the consequences of respiratory depression (Huf *et al*, 2011).

In the UK, midazolam injection is unlicensed for intramuscular use: only intravenous administration is licensed (Roche, 2008), which would be inappropriate for rapid tranquillisation.

Midazolam: buccal and sublingual

Buccal and sublingual midazolam have been studied in a number of populations and scenarios, notably as an emergency anti-epileptic in paediatrics and intellectual disabilities as an alternative to rectal diazepam, where the route of administration is a key feature (Sweetman, 2009). It has also been used for rapid tranquillisation in adult psychiatric patients (Taylor *et al*, 2008).

Sublingual midazolam is quickly absorbed, including via the buccal mucosa, and gives high bioavailability (about 75%) and reliable plasma concentrations (Schwagmeier *et al*, 1998). However, there is a minimal role for the use of buccal or sublingual midazolam in rapid tranquillisation, as it requires the patient to agree to taking an oral formulation (Taylor *et al*, 2009). In such cases, lorazepam tablets, which are licensed and widely available, would be a more familiar choice.

49

Other agents available outside of the UK

Several other parenteral agents are licensed for rapid tranquillisation and available outside of the UK.

Clonazepam

Only licensed in the UK for intravenous administration in status epilepticus. It is a long-acting benzodiazepine and, like diazepam, has active metabolites, therefore there is a risk of accumulation. It has a higher risk of profound hypotension than lorazepam, and may be used in countries where intramuscular lorazepam is not available.

Droperidol

Remains available in the USA but production was discontinued in the UK in 2001 (Current Problems in Pharmacovigilance, 2001) following the conclusion in a meta-analysis that it increased the risk of QT interval prolongation (cardiac repolarisation) in a dose-dependent manner (Reilly et al, 2000).

Loxapine

A typical antipsychotic available in formulations for oral and intramuscular administration in several countries (excluding the UK). It has been licensed in the USA in a formulation for inhalation from a breath-actuated device for rapid tranquillisation. It has demonstrated superior efficacy to placebo with a quick onset of action (Allen et al, 2011; Lesem et al, 2011).

Perphenazine

A phenothiazine antipsychotic, similar to chlorpromazine, its intramuscular use is limited by its propensity to cause hypotension, sedation and EPS.

Ziprasidone

Both the oral and intramuscular injection formulations of this atypical antipsychotic are unlikely to be licensed in the UK, although it has been available in the USA since 2001. There is increasing clinical experience with the intramuscular injection for rapid tranquillisation (Brook et al, 2000; Baldacara et al, 2011), including in children and adolescents (Khan & Mican, 2006; Barzman et al, 2007), older adults (Kohen et al, 2005; Barak et al, 2006) and the medically unwell (Martel et al, 2005).

Unrecommended agents in the UK

In addition to the above, the following agents are available in the UK but are not recommended for rapid tranquillisation: zuclopenthixol acetate, intramuscular diazepam, parental chlorpromazine, amylobarbitone (or 'amobarbital'), paraldehyde and intramuscular depot antipsychotics (National Institute for Health and Clinical Excellence, 2005; Ahmed et al, 2010).

Familiarity with responsibilities and processes in rapid tranquillisation

It is strongly recommended that all staff involved in the prescribing and administration of medicines for rapid tranquillisation should be familiar with the practical arrangements and responsibilities in this regard.

Doctors who prescribe rapid tranquillisation should (Royal College of Psychiatrists, 1998; National Institute for Health and Clinical Excellence, 2005):

- be familiar with the properties of benzodiazepines and their antagonists, antipsychotics, antimuscarinics and antihistamines
- be able to assess the risks associated with rapid tranquillisation, particularly when the patient is highly aroused and may have been misusing drugs, may be dehydrated or physically ill
- understand the cardiovascular effects of the acute administration of the tranquillising medications and the need to titrate the dose
- recognise the importance of nursing in the recovery position
- recognise the importance of monitoring pulse, blood pressure and respiration
- be familiar and trained in the use of resuscitation equipment
- undertake regular resuscitation training
- understand the importance of maintaining an unobstructed airway.

Seeking advice in rapid tranquillisation

Any member of the professional team caring for a patient who requires rapid tranquillisation should seek the advice of a senior colleague or a member of another profession (e.g. pharmacist, senior nurse or matron) at any stage in the rapid tranquillisation process if they are at all unsure about the intended treatment plan. This may include situations when a patient does not respond as expected to the prescribed doses, if the maximum BNF dose has been given yet there is a clinical need for further pharmacological management, if the prescription is unclear/illegible, or if the clinician is unfamiliar with the use of the prescribed medication (either formulation or dose).

Monitoring post rapid tranquillisation

After rapid tranquillisation has been administered, it is essential to check the patient's physical well-being. If the patient has refused oral medication and as a result has been given intramuscular injections, this may have involved physically restraining the patient. The injection of one or more medicines into a person who is physically stressed by the restraint process can lead to adverse physical sequelae.

The National Institute for Health and Clinical Excellence (2005) recommends that 'blood pressure, pulse, temperature and respiratory rate and hydration should be recorded regularly' post rapid tranquillisation. However, there are no national standards or recommendations on the specific intervals or duration of physical monitoring parameters post rapid tranquillisation, and local trust guidelines vary considerably in their detail and recommended frequencies (Innes & Iyeke, 2012). In view of the relatively high risk of cardiac arrhythmias associated with the use of haloperidol in particular, some trusts also monitor the electrocardiogram (ECG) and find this measure more practicable than trying to measure blood pressure in a resistive patient.

The recommendations in Table 5.1 are pragmatic suggestions for monitoring vital signs, balancing the need of monitoring the patient's health to ensure physical safety with the realities of nursing distressed and acutely disturbed patients.

Pulse oximeters should be available and staff should be familiar with their use. Additionally, ECG machines should be available at all sites where parenteral haloperidol is given, as the Summary of Product Characteristics for intramuscular haloperidol recommends that prior to treatment a baseline ECG is conducted in all patients, especially in the elderly and those with a positive personal or family history of cardiac disease or abnormal findings on cardiac clinical examination.

The above parameters and the patient's general level of consciousness should be monitored and recorded regularly until the patient becomes active again. Judgement of the patient's relative level of activity/inactivity should be based on a clinical assessment on a case-by-case basis. If nursing staff are unable to monitor any of these parameters, the reasons for such omissions must also be documented.

It is recommended that measurements should be documented on a specific rapid tranquillisation observation record form.

In circumstances where the patient is at a higher risk, more frequent and intensive monitoring by appropriately trained staff is required and should be recorded. Particular attention should be paid to the patient's respiratory effort, airway and level of consciousness:

Table 5.1 Recommendations for monitoring vital signs

Route of administration	Frequency of measurements
Oral only	If patient is inactive the nursing staff must use their clinical judgement on the level of monitoring required, taking account of risk factors
Intramuscular	Every 15 min for the first hour, then hourly for 4 h or until the patient becomes active again. More frequent monitoring may be instigated following the clinical judgement of the nurse or doctor and discussion with the team

- if the patient appears to be or is asleep/sedated
- if the BNF limit or Summary of Product Characteristics is exceeded
- if an older adult's mobility is affected, or they are at high risk of falls
- where the patient has been recently using illicit substances or alcohol
- where the patient has a relevant medical disorder or concurrently prescribed medication.

Risks and complications associated with rapid tranquillisation

There are specific risks associated with the different classes of medications that are used in rapid tranquillisation. Staff using these medicines should be aware of them (National Institute for Health and Clinical Excellence, 2005). Table 5.2 lists some common and some serious adverse effects following the administration of rapid tranquillisation, and the recommended management.

When prescribing medication for rapid tranquillisation, the specific properties of the individual medications should be taken into consideration; when combinations are used, risks may be compounded.

As mentioned earlier, the use of intravenous and high doses of antipsychotics is of concern because of the potential to increase QT interval and the associated risk of tachyarrhythmias. Respiratory depression (by accumulated doses of benzodiazepines, and in the past, barbituates) or laryngeal stridor, causing stridor and hypoxia, are postulated causes for other unexplained sudden deaths of acutely disturbed patients prescribed medication.

Sedation is a risk factor for venous thromboembolic disease (National Institute for Health and Clinical Excellence, 2010a), particularly in patients who are obese, dehydrated, have comorbid cardiac disease or diabetes, or are taking oestrogen-containing contraceptives or hormone replacement therapy. Patients should be assessed using the risk assessment for venous thromboembolism (National Institute for Health and Clinical Excellence, 2010b).

Circumstances for special care

Extra care should be taken when implementing rapid tranquillisation in the following circumstances:

- the presence of congenital prolonged QTc syndromes;
- the concurrent prescription or use of other medication that lengthens QTc intervals both directly and indirectly;
- prolonged QTc interval is a marker for cardiac arrhythmia: potential cardiorespiratory collapse and physical exertion, stress, illicit drug use (ecstasy and cannabis, and possibly other illicit drugs) and metabolic factors are risk factors;
- the presence of certain disorders affecting metabolism, such as hypo-/ hyperthermia, stress and extreme emotions, and extreme physical exertion.

Table 5.2 Common or serious adverse effects following rapid tranquillisation and recommended management

Complication	Symptoms/signs	Management
Acute dystonia	Severe painful muscular stiffness	Procyclidine 5–10 mg intramuscularly
Hypotension	Fall in blood pressure (orthostatic or <50 mmHg diastolic)	Lie patient flat and raise legs – tilt bed head down. Monitor closely. Seek medical advice
Neuroleptic malignant syndrome	Increasing temperature, fluctuating blood pressure, muscular rigidity, confusion/fluctuating or altered consciousness	Neuroleptic malignant syndrome is a potentially serious, even fatal, side-effect. Medical advice should be sought immediately Withhold antipsychotics Monitor closely (temperature, blood pressure, pulse) Liaise with general medical team
Arrhythmias	Slow (<50/min), irregular or impalpable pulse	Monitor vital observations and electrocardiogram and liaise with general medical team immediately May require immediate defibrillation
Respiratory depression	Reducing respiratory rate, reducing consciousness	Give oxygen, and place the patient in the recovery position, instigating measures for basic life support If indicated, an oropharyngeal/nasopharyngeal airway should be inserted and the patient mechanically ventilated. This should only be undertaken when appropriately qualified and skilled staff are available If respiratory rate drops below 10 breaths/min, seek medical advice. If the patient has received benzodiazepines, give flumazenil: • 200 mcg intravenously over 15 s • if consciousness not resumed within 60 s, give 100 mcg over 10 s • repeat at 60-second intervals; maximum dose 1 mg/24 h Continue to monitor after respiratory rate returns to normal. Flumazenil has a shorter duration of action than many benzodiazepines so repeated doses may be required. Patients may become agitated or anxious on waking. Flumazenil is best avoided in patients with epilepsy – start mechanical ventilation instead

Older adults and rapid tranquillisation

In mental health service structures, patients aged 65 years and older are commonly cared for in separate services to working-age adults, and may be referred to as 'older adults'. As with all other medication, when prescribing rapid tranquillisation medication for patients in this population, their age should not be the only deciding factor when determining a regimen. The physical fitness of the individual must be considered. Particular care should be given to coexisting medical states and prescribed medication, the risk of accumulation of sedatives and the possibility of delirium. Both antipsychotics and benzodiazepines may affect mobility and increase the risk of falls. Patients should be monitored for signs of impaired mobility and unsteadiness. Older people are at increased risk of venous thromboembolic disease (National Institute for Health and Clinical Excellence, 2010).

The NICE guidelines (National Collaborating Centre for Mental Health, 2007) recommend that:

> 'If rapid tranquillisation is needed, a combination of [intramuscular] IM haloperidol and IM lorazepam should be considered. IM diazepam and IM chlorpromazine are not recommended for the management of behaviour that challenges in people with dementia. If using IM haloperidol (or any other IM conventional antipsychotic) for behavioural control, healthcare professionals should monitor closely for dystonia and other extrapyramidal side effects. If side effects become distressing, especially in acute dystonic reactions, the use of anticholinergic agents should be considered. If using anticholinergic agents, healthcare professionals should monitor for deteriorating cognitive function' (p. 32).

Lorazepam remains the first medicine of choice in this population (oral or intramuscular route), but if two or more parenteral doses or $\geq 2\,mg$ lorazepam during one episode are required, junior staff should seek advice from senior colleagues. Older adults may have poorer muscle perfusion than younger patients, which may produce erratic absorption of intramuscularly administered medicines into the blood stream. Therefore a longer interval should be allowed between intramuscular doses (at least 1 h).

The Medicines and Healthcare products Regulatory Agency recommended that olanzapine and risperidone are not to be used in the treatment of behavioural symptoms of dementia, due to the increased risk of stroke (Duff, 2004). However, from observational data, the European Pharmacovigilance Working Party (2005) concluded that the likelihood of cerebrovascular adverse events associated with the use of conventional antipsychotics in patients with dementia was not significantly different from that of olanzapine and risperidone. Therefore it is recommended that antipsychotics for rapid tranquillisation are only prescribed to patients with dementia or a history of cerebrovascular events after careful consideration and where lorazepam alone is insufficient or inappropriate. This decision to prescribe antipsychotics for rapid tranquilisation should be documented in the notes, with the rationale clearly recorded.

55

Patients under 18 years of age and rapid tranquillisation

Although the evidence base for the use of specific pharmacological therapies in the general psychiatric population is not very rigorous and is based on relatively small numbers, data in children and adolescents are even more so and predominantly collected from settings outside the UK (Sorrentino, 2004). When using medicines for rapid tranquillisation in children and young people aged under 18 years, the same good principles (pp. 35–36) still apply, in addition to the following factors.

As with all patients receiving rapid tranquillisation medication, a child/adolescent must be informed that medication is going to be given and must be given the opportunity at any stage to accept oral medication voluntarily. In children/adolescents who are not Gillick competent, parents/carers should be informed of the situation and their consent sought for such treatment. It is good practice to inform both the child/adolescent and their parents/carers.

When treating children and adolescents, even greater effort should be made to avoid the use of typical antipsychotics, as this patient group is more likely to be antipsychotic-naive and sensitive to EPS. Therefore if oral treatment is accepted, risperidone (tablets or liquid or dispersible tablet) may be more appropriate (Joint Formulary Committee, 2011; Paediatric Formulary Committee, 2011). In children with moderate, severe or profound intellectual disability and/or epilepsy, even smaller doses of risperidone should be considered (Einfeld, 2001; Allington-Smith, 2006).

As there is a higher incidence of disinhibition or paradoxical reactions with benzodiazepines in children compared with adults, this should be borne in mind if using lorazepam. If haloperidol injection is used, consider also giving prophylactic procyclidine because of the higher incidence of EPS. Other medicine options for this population include the sedating antihistamine alimemazine (previously called trimeprazine), given orally as a tablet or liquid (Joint Formulary Committee 2011; Paediatric Formulary Committee, 2011).

In younger children, the formulation of the medicines may become even more pertinent and guide the choice of agent (Paediatric Formulary Committee, 2011). Several of the above medicines are available in liquid formulations or as dispersible tablets. It should also be noted that many of these medications are unlicensed in this age group for this indication.

Pregnancy and rapid tranquillisation

According to the NICE (2007) guidelines on antenatal and postnatal mental health, a pregnant woman requiring rapid tranquillisation should be treated in accordance with the 2005 NICE guidelines on the short-term management of disturbed behaviour, with the following provisos:

- following rapid tranquillisation a pregnant woman should not be put in seclusion

- restraint procedures should be adapted to avoid possible harm to the fetus
- the woman's care during the perinatal period should be managed in close collaboration with a paediatrician and an anaesthetist.

The National Institute for Health and Care Excellence also recommends that the antipsychotic or a benzodiazepine used should be one with a short half-life; however, this does not differ from the general recommendations where lorazepam (a short-acting benzodiazepine) is considered as first-line treatment.

Starting regular antipsychotic treatment after rapid tranquillisation

After rapid tranquillisation has been given, the continuation of medication in the medium to longer term is clearly indicated in patients with an established psychiatric illness that would usually be treated by medication (e.g. a patient with a diagnosis of schizophrenia who has relapsed following cessation of antipsychotic treatment in the community). A similar scenario in a patient with bipolar affective disorder might indicate the need for the longer-term use of mood-stabilising medication (antipsychotic and/or mood stabiliser(s)).

In patients who do not have a mental illness that would usually require medium- to long-term prescribing, the short-term prescribing of regular medication after rapid tranquillisation may still be indicated. For example, a highly aroused patient with a diagnosis of personality disorder may require the use of regular anxiolytic medication for a few days or weeks following rapid tranquillisation until their condition has stabilised and the risk of further violence significantly reduced.

The final choice of agent and the formulation and route of administration should be guided by factors such as the patient's medication history, current medication regime, patient's preference including advanced directive if made, their response and tolerance to treatment to date, and consideration as to whether they are willing to take oral medication prescribed as tablets, or whether liquid or dispersible medication prescribed under supervision, or a depot, is indicated.

Ethnicity and rapid tranquillisation

There have been concerns that African–Caribbean patients may be given rapid tranquillisation more often that other ethnic groups. Various explanations have been postulated for this such as institutional racism, including the possibility of late presentation and/or racial bias in clinicians' perceptions of dangerousness of patients.

The NICE guidelines (2005) concluded: 'There is insufficient evidence to assess whether African Caribbean service users are given rapid tranquillisation more often than service users from other ethnic backgrounds' (p. 59) and 'it is therefore not possible to ascertain if different cultural groups exhibit higher or lower levels of disturbed/violent behaviour than other groups' (p. 58).

However, it remains the responsibility of all staff to ensure that if concerns emerge regarding the inappropriate use of medication, including rapid tranquillisation, in patients from an ethnic minority, or indeed any patient, they are immediately passed on to the trust management for appropriate action.

Monitoring and audit of rapid tranquillisation

The use of rapid tranquillisation, particularly when the ability to give or withhold consent is limited, must be subject to frequent and careful review with central audit and monitoring by trust/unit management.

All psychiatric units should have policies and procedures for the use of emergency medication, and aspects of practice with regard to rapid tranquillisation should be carefully recorded and regularly audited.

Pro re nata (p.r.n.) medication

Commonly, in-patient prescription charts have the facility to prescribe medicines p.r.n. This important 'provision' enables doctors to prescribe specific medicines that nurses may administer at their clinical discretion.

Medicines such as lorazepam, haloperidol and procyclidine (both orally and intramuscularly) are often prescribed on the p.r.n. section of in-patient prescription charts in many acute psychiatric wards. However, such p.r.n. prescriptions, in addition to the regularly prescribed psychotropics, may enable the administration of greater than BNF maximum doses (Baker, 2008) and encourage polypharmacy if patients are already prescribed other regular psychotropics from the same group (e.g. antipsychotics), which may put the patient at clinical risk. It is therefore important that the indication and use of p.r.n. medication prescribed is clearly stated and regularly reviewed.

References

Ahmed, U., Jones, H. & Adams C. E. (2010) Chlorpromazine for psychosis induced aggression or agitation. *Cochrane Database of Systematic Reviews*, 4, CD007445.

Alexander, J., Tharyan, P., Adams, C., *et al* (2004) Rapid tranquillisation of violent or agitated patients in psychiatric emergency setting. Pragmatic randomised trial of intramuscular lorazepam v. haloperidol plus promethazine. *British Journal of Psychiatry*, 185, 63–69.

Allen, M. H., Currier, G. W., Carpenter, D., *et al* (2005) Treatment of behavioural emergencies (Expert consensus guideline series). *Journal of Psychiatric Practice*, 11 (suppl. 1), 1–108.

Allen, M. H., Feifal, D., Lesem, M. D., *et al* (2011) Efficacy and safety of loxapine for inhalation in the treatment of agitation in patients with schizophrenia: a randomized, double-blind, placebo-controlled trial. *Journal of Clinical Psychiatry*, 7, 1313–1321.

Allington-Smith, P. (2006) Mental health of children with learning disabilities. *Advances in Psychiatric Treatment*, **12**, 130–138.

Andrezina, R., Josiassen, R. C., Marcus, R. N., *et al* (2006) Intramuscular aripiprazole for the treatment of acute agitation in patients with schizophrenia or schizoaffective disorder: a double-blind, placebo-controlled comparison with intramuscular haloperidol. *Psychopharmacology*, **188**, 281–292.

Applebaum, P. S., Robbins, P. C. & Monahan, J. (2000) Violence and delusions: data from the McArthur Violence Risk Assessment Study. *American Journal of Psychiatry*, **157**, 566–572.

Aupperle, P. (2006) Management of aggression, agitation, and psychosis in dementia: focus on atypical antipsychotics. *American Journal of Alzheimer's Disease and Other Dementias*, **21**, 101–108.

Baker, J. A. (2008) A best-evidence synthesis review of the administration of psychotropic pro re nata (PRN) medication in in-patient mental health settings. *Journal of Clinical Nursing*, **17**, 1122–1131.

Baldacara, L., Sanches, M., Cordeiro, D. C., *et al* (2011) Rapid tranquilization for agitated patients in emergency psychiatric rooms: a randomized trial of olanzapine, ziprasidone, haloperidol plus promethazine, haloperidol plus midazolam and haloperidol alone. *Revista Brasileira de Psiquiatria*, **33**, 30–39.

Ballard, C. G., Birks, J. & Waite, J. (2006) Atypical antipsychotics for aggression and psychosis in Alzheimer disease. *Cochrane Database of Systematic Reviews*, **1**, CD003476.

Barak, Y., Mazeh, D., Plopski, I., *et al* (2006) Intramuscular ziprasidone treatment of acute psychotic agitation in elderly patients with schizophrenia. *American Journal of Geriatric Psychiatry*, **14**, 629–633.

Barzman, D. H., DelBello, M. P., Forrester, J. J., *et al* (2007) A retrospective chart review of intramuscular ziprasidone for agitation in children and adolescents on psychiatric units: Prospective studies are needed. *Journal of Child and Adolescent Psychopharmacology*, **17**, 503–509.

Battaglia, J. (2005) Pharmacological management of acute agitation. *Drugs*, **65**, 1207–1222.

Belgamwar, R. B. & Fenton, M. (2005) Olanzapine IM or velotabs for acutely disturbed/agitated people with suspected serious mental illness. *Cochrane Database of Systematic Reviews*, **2**, CD003729.

Brieden, T., Ujeyl, M. & Naber, D. (2002) Psychopharmacological treatment of aggression in schizophrenic patients. *Pharmacopsychiatry*, **35**, 83–89.

Broadstock, M. (2001) The effectiveness and safety of drug treatment for urgent sedation in psychiatric emergencies: a critical appraisal of the literature. *New Zealand Health Technology Assessment*, **4**, Number 1.

Brook, S., Lucey, J. V. & Gunn, K. P. (2000) Intramuscular haloperidol in the treatment of acute psychosis. *Journal of Clinical Psychiatry*, **61**, 933–941.

Caine, E. D. (2006) Clinical perspective on atypical antipsychotics for treatment of agitation. *Journal of Clinical Psychiatry*, **67** (suppl. 10), 22–31.

Care Quality Commission (2008) *Guidance for SOADS: Consent for Treatment and the SOAD Role under the Revised Mental Health Act*. CQC.

Chengappa, K. N., Vasile, J., Levine, J., *et al* (2002) Clozapine: its impact on aggressive behaviour among patients in a state psychiatric hospital. *Schizophrenia Research*, **53**, 1–6.

Current Problems in Pharmacovigilance (2001) QT interval prolongation with antipsychotics. *Current Problems in Pharmacovigilance*, **27**, 4.

Duff, G. (2004) Atypical antipsychotic drugs and stroke. Committee on Safety of Medicines (http://www.mhra.gov.uk/home/groups/pl-p/documents/websiteresources/con019488.pdf).

Einfeld, S. L. (2001) Systematic management approach to pharmacotherapy for people with learning disabilities. *Advances in Psychiatric Treatment*, **7**, 43–49.

Eli Lilly (2004) *Important Safety Information: Reported Serious Adverse Events following use of Zyprexa Intramuscular (28 September)*. Eli Lilly (http://www.palliativedrugs.com/download/SafetyLetterzyprexa.pdf).

Eli Lilly (2009) Zyprexa powder for solution for injection. Electronic Medicines Compendium.

European Pharmacovigilance Working Party (2005) *Antipsychotics and Cerebrovascular Accident*. European Medicines Agency.

Gillies, D., Beck, A., McCloud, A., *et al* (2010) Benzodiazepines for psychosis-induced aggression or agitation. *Cochrane Database of Systematic Reviews*, **4**, CD003079.

Goedhard, L. E., Stolker, J. J., Heerdink, E. R., *et al* (2006) Pharmacotherapy for the treatment of aggressive behaviour in general adult psychiatry: a systematic review. *Journal of Clinical Psychiatry*, **67**, 1013–1024.

Gordon, H. & Grubin, D. (2004) Psychiatric aspects of the assessment and treatment of sex offenders. *Advances in Psychiatric Treatment*, **10**, 73–80.

Hassaballa, H. A. & Balk, R. A. (2003*a*) Torsade de pointes associated with the administration of intravenous haloperidol. *American Journal of Therapeutics*, **10**, 58–60.

Hassaballa, H. A. & Balk, R. A. (2003*b*) Torsade de pointes associated with the administration of intravenous haloperidol: a review of the literature and practical guidelines for use. *Expert Opinion on Drug Safety*, **2**, 543–547.

Hsu, W.-Y., Huang, S-S., Lee, B-S., *et al* (2010) Comparison of intramuscular olanzapine, orally disintegrating olanzapine tablets, oral risperidone solution, and intramuscular haloperidol in the management of acute agitation in an acute care psychiatric ward in Taiwan. *Journal of Clinical Psychopharmacology*, **30**, 230–234.

Huf, G., Coutinho, E. S. & Adams, C. E. (2007) Rapid tranquillisation in psychiatric emergency settings in Brazil: pragmatic randomised controlled trial of intramuscular haloperidol versus intramuscular haloperidol plus promethazine. *BMJ*, **335**, 869–875.

Huf, G., Alexander, J., Allen, M. H., *et al* (2011) Haloperidol plus promethazine for psychosis-induced aggression. *Cochrane Database of Systematic Reviews*, **3**, CD005146.

Innes, J. & Iyeke, L. (2012) A review of the practice and position of monitoring in today's rapid tranquilisation protocol. *Journal of Psychiatric Intensive Care*, **8**, 15–24.

Isbister, G. K., Calver, L. A., Page, C. B., *et al* (2010) Randomized controlled trial of intramuscular droperidol versus midazolam for violence and acute behavioural disturbance: the DORM study. *Annals of Emergency Medicine*, **56**, 392–401.

Jacobson, R. R. (1997) Commentary: Aggression and impulsivity after head injury. *Advances in Psychiatric Treatment*, **3**, 160–163.

Joint Formulary Committee (2011) *British National Formulary 62: September 2011*. BMJ Group and Pharmaceutical Press.

Khan, S. S. & Mican, L. M. (2006) A naturalistic evaluation of intramuscular ziprasidone versus olanzapine for the management of acute agitation and aggression in children and adolescents. *Journal of Child and Adolescent Psychopharmacology*, **16**, 671–677.

Kohen, I., Preval, H., Southard, R., *et al* (2005) Naturalistic study of intramuscular ziprasidone versus conventional agents in agitated elderly patients: retrospective findings from a psychiatric emergency service. *American Journal of Geriatric Pharmacotherapy*, **3**, 240–245.

Krakowski, M. I., Czobor, P., Citrome, L., *et al* (2006) Atypical antipsychotic agents in the treatment of violent patients with schizophrenia and schizoaffective disorder. *Archives of General Psychiatry*, **63**, 622–629.

Krakowski, M. I., Czobor, P. & Nolan, K. A. (2008) Atypical antipsychotics, neurocognitive deficits, and aggression in schizophrenic patients. *Journal of Clinical Psychopharmacology*, **28**, 485–493.

Krakowski, M. I. & Czobor, P. (2011) Neurocognitive impairment limits the response to treatment of aggression with antipsychotic agents. *Schizophrenia Bulletin*, **37** (suppl. 1), 311–312.

Kraus, J. E. & Sheitman, M. D. (2005) Clozapine reduces violent behaviour in hetero-geneous diagnostic groups. *Journal of Neuropsychiatry and Clinical Neurosciences*, **17**, 36–44.

Lesem, M. D., Tran-Johnson, T. K., Reinsenberg, R. A., *et al* (2011) Rapid acute treatment of agitation in individuals with schizophrenia: multicentre, randomised, placebo-controlled study of inhaled loxapine. *British Journal of Psychiatry*, **198**, 51–58.

Marder, S. R. (2006) A review of agitation in mental illness: treatment guidelines and current therapies. *Journal of Clinical Psychiatry*, **67** (suppl. 10), 13–21.

Martel, M., Sterzinger, A., Miner, J., *et al* (2005) Management of acute undifferentiated agitation in the emergency department: a randomized double-blind trial of droperidol, ziprasidone, and midazolam. *Academic Emergency Medicine*, **12**, 1167–1172.

National Institute for Health and Clinical Excellence (2003) *Guidance on the Use of Electroconvulsive Therapy* (Technology Appraisal TA59). NICE.

National Institute for Health and Clinical Excellence (2005) *Violence: The Short-term Management of Disturbed/Violent Behavior in In-patient Psychiatric Settings and Emergency Departments* (Clinical Guideline CG25). NICE.

National Collaborating Centre for Mental Health (2007) *Dementia: A NICE–SCIE Guideline on Supporting People with Dementia and their Carers in Health and Social Care* (National Clinical Practice Guideline CG42). British Psychological Society & Gaskell.

National Institute for Health and Clinical Excellence (2007) *Antenatal and Postnatal Mental Health: Clinical Management and Service Guidance* (Clinical Guideline CG45). NICE.

National Institute for Health and Clinical Excellence (2009*a*) *Borderline Personality Disorder: The NICE Guideline on Treatment and Management* (Clinical Guideline CG78). The British Psychological Society & The Royal College of Psychiatrists.

National Institute for Health and Clinical Excellence (2009*b*) *Antisocial Personality Disorder: Treatment, Management and Prevention* (Clinical Guideline CG77). NICE.

National Institute for Health and Clinical Excellence (2009*c*) *Depression: The Treatment and Management of Depression in Adults* (Clinical Guideline CG90). NICE.

National Institute for Health and Clinical Excellence (2010*a*) *Venous Thromboembolism: Reducing the Risk* (Clinical Guideline CG92). NICE.

National Institute for Health and Clinical Excellence (2010*b*) *Venous Thromboembolism: Reducing the Risk Quick Reference Guide*. NICE.

Nobay, F., Simon, B. C., Levitt, A., *et al* (2004) A prospective, double-blind, randomized trial of midazolam versus haloperidol versus lorazepam in the chemical restraint of violent and severely agitated patients. *Academic Emergency Medicine*, **11**, 744–749.

Oakley, C., Hynes, F. & Clark, T. (2009) Mood disorders and violence: a new focus. *Advances in Psychiatric Treatment*, **15**, 263–270.

Paediatric Formulary Committee (2011) *BNF for Children 2011–2012*. Pharmaceutical Press.

Parker, C. & Khwaja, M. (2011) What is new in rapid tranquillisation? *Journal of Psychiatric Intensive Care*, **7**, 91–101.

Raveendran, N. S., Tharyan, P., Alexander, J., *et al* (2007) Rapid tranquillisation in psychiatric emergency settings in India: pragmatic randomised controlled trial of intramuscular olanzapine versus intramuscular haloperidol plus promethazine. *BMJ*, **335**, 865–872.

Reilly, J. G., Ayis, S. A., Ferrier, I. N., *et al* (2000) QTc-interval abnormalities and psychotropic drug therapy in psychiatric patients. *Lancet*, **355**, 1048–1052.

Roche (2008) Hypnovel 10mg/2ml solution for injection. Electronic Medicines Compendium.

Royal College of Psychiatrists (1998) *Management of Imminent Violence: Clinical Practice Guidelines to Support Mental Health Services* (Occasional Paper OP41). Royal College of Psychiatrists.

Royal College of Psychiatrists (2006) *Consensus Statement on High-dose Antipsychotic Medication (Council Report CR138)*. Royal College of Psychiatrists.

Schwagmeier, R., Alincic, S. & Striebel, H. W. (1998) Midazolam pharmacokinetics following intravenous and buccal administration. *British Journal of Clinical Pharmacology*, **46**, 203–206.

Soloff, P. H. (1998) Algorithms for pharmacological treatment of personality dimensions. Symptom-specific treatments for cognitive-perceptual, affective, and impulsive-behavioural dysregulation. *Bulletin of the Menninger Clinic*, **62**, 195–214.

Sorrentino, A. (2004) Chemical restraints for the agitated, violent or psychotic paediatric patients in the emergency department: controversies and recommendations. *Current Opinion in Paediatrics*, **16**, 201–205.

Swanson, J. W., Swartz, M. S., Van Dorn, R. A., *et al* (2008) Comparison of antipsychotic medication effects on reducing violence in people with schizophrenia. *British Journal of Psychiatry*, **193**, 37–43.

Sweetman, S. (2009) *Martindale: The Complete Drug Reference*. MedicinesComplete (http://www.medicinescomplete.com/mc/martindale/current/).

Taylor, D., Okocha, C., Paton, C., *et al* (2008) Buccal midazolam for agitation on psychiatric intensive care wards. *International Journal of Psychiatry in Clinical Practice*, **12**, 309–311.

Taylor, D., Paton, C. & Kapur, S. (2009) *Maudsley Prescribing Guidelines, Tenth Edition*. Informa Healthcare.

Tharyan, P. & C. E. Adams (2005) *Electroconvulsive Therapy for Schizophrenia (Review)*. Wiley.

Tran-Johnson, T. K., Sack, D. A., Marcus, R. N., *et al* (2007) Efficacy and safety of intramuscular aripiprazole in patients with acute agitation: a randomized double blind, placebo-controlled trial. *Journal of Clinical Psychiatry*, **68**, 111–119.

TREC Collaborative Group (2003) Rapid tranquillisation for agitated patients in psychiatric rooms: a randomised trial of midazolam versus haloperidol plus promethazine. *BMJ*, **327**, 708–711.

Tyrer, P. & Bateman, A. W. (2004) Drug treatment for personality disorders. *Advances in Psychiatric Treatment*, **10**, 389–398.

Volavka, J., Czobor, P., Nolan, K., *et al* (2004) Overt aggression and psychotic symptoms in patients with schizophrenia treated with clozapine, olanzapine, risperidone, or haloperidol. *Journal of Clinical Psychopharmacology*, **24**, 225–228.

Waite, J. & Easton, A. (eds) *(2013) The Ect Handbook* (3rd edn) (College Report CR176). RCPsych Publications.

Wright, P., Birkett, M., David, S. R., *et al* (2001) Double blind, placebo-controlled comparison of intramuscular olanzapine and intramuscular haloperidol in the treatment of acute agitation in schizophrenia. *American Journal of Psychiatry*, **158**, 1149–1151.

Zimbroff, D. L., Marcus, R. N., Manos, G., *et al* (2007) Management of acute agitation in patients with bipolar disorder: efficacy and safety of intramuscular aripiprazole. *Journal of Clinical Psychopharmacology*, **27**, 171–176.

CHAPTER 6

Post-incident management

Laura Garrod, Masum Khwaja and Ian Cumming

Aggression can be expressed in many forms, ranging from a service user raising their voice during an argument to an unprovoked attack involving a weapon. Evidence suggests that all types of aggressive behaviour can pose a threat to the physical and psychological health of the individual(s) involved (Wykes, 1994).

Not all incidents can be prevented, so it is important to have specific procedures in place for responding to incidents. Employers are required to ensure there are systems to support staff affected by an incident under the Health and Safety at Work etc Act 1974.

Mental health service providers should have systems in place with appropriately skilled staff to ensure that a menu of post-incident support and review are available and take place within a culture of learning to make services safer (National Institute for Mental Health in England, 2004). A senior member of staff should coordinate the activities of others post incident. Involving senior members of a team emphasises that incidents of violence are taken seriously.

Post-incident review

Post-incident review is broadly defined as an evaluation of incident response used to identify and correct weaknesses, as well as determine strengths and promulgate them. The establishment of facts surrounding an incident should be undertaken as part of a timely factual 'debrief' and the incident reported according to local organisational guidelines. The extent of the post-incident review will depend on the seriousness of the incident.

Psychological debriefing may be defined as a set of procedures including counselling and the giving of information aimed at preventing psychological morbidity and aiding recovery after a traumatic event (Kenardy, 2000). The process of debriefing has two functions: to establish factual details and to provide emotional support. Separating 'technical' and 'emotional' debriefings may help ensure that people can contribute to the factual investigation of an incident while receiving emotional support.

Although debriefing has not been shown to prevent future psychological distress (Raphael *et al*, 1985; Rose *et al*, 2009), the experience of workers in the field is that victims (patient, staff, carers) are grateful for the opportunity to express feelings and achieve some understanding of what happened (McIvor *et al*, 1997; Bonner & Wellman, 2010), and staff find it helpful to be brought together in a post-incident review meeting to discuss what happened.

A post-incident review should take place as soon as possible after the incident and ideally before the end of a shift or working day. If this cannot be achieved the review must be conducted within 72 h.

Appropriate support, including ongoing individual post-incident review sessions, should also be made available as required.

The post-incident review should address what happened immediately before and during the incident; consider any contributing factors, each person's role in the incident, how they felt during the incident, how they feel at the time of the review, how they may feel in the near future, and what can be done to address their concerns. The aims of the post-incident review is to learn from the incident, assure those involved that their reaction is normal, that the care team's cohesiveness is not affected, to anticipate reactions as time goes on, to reduce discomfort and tension, to provide immediate and continuing support and to seek reconciliation of the therapeutic relationship between staff, service users and their carers.

It is also important that a separate post-incident review meeting or debrief is arranged for service users as well as for carers and visitors where appropriate as soon as it is practically possible. During incidents, service users often feel vulnerable, frightened, confused and exposed. These experiences can exacerbate symptoms of mental illness or generally unsettle service users. It is helpful if some staff involved in the incident assist in facilitating the debrief so that service users, carers and visitors can experience some consistency and see staff coping.

The following groups should be considered for inclusion in the review:

- staff involved in the incident
- service users involved in the incident
- carers and family where appropriate
- other service users who witnessed the incident
- independent advocates
- local security management specialists.

The rules for de-briefing are:

- make sure everyone involved is invited and everyone who wants to attend can
- allow adequate time for preparation and follow-up
- participation is voluntary
- the meeting is strictly confidential
- attendants do not have to say anything

- there is no rank, everyone is equal
- this is not a criticism or investigation
- this is not counselling
- techniques such as offering insight, probing or being non-directive should be avoided
- expect anger to be expressed.

Post-incident action

Perpetrator

A medical review of the patient's mental and physical state should take place within 2 h (National Institute for Mental Health in England, 2002). The review should include consideration of the Mental Health Act status of the patient, the observation level, and the setting for further treatment. Risk assessment and care plan documentation should be updated.

Following each intervention for the short-term management of disturbed/violent behaviour, it should be established whether the service user understands why the intervention took place. They may be upset by the incident or how it was managed, or frightened about the consequences for them, and they should therefore be given the opportunity to discuss the incident from their perspective. Where possible, this should be carried out by a staff member who was not directly involved in the intervention. The discussion should be documented in the service user's notes.

Whether to pursue criminal proceedings is discussed below.

Victim

Immediate first aid and medical treatment should be given to the injured person(s) where appropriate. A member of staff should be identified to stay with the injured person(s) until medial assistance is available.

It is important that victims know their rights, for example the right to report a violent attack to the police. The individual's manager should discuss the issue of prosecution and offer to accompany the relevant service user(s) or staff member(s) to police if necessary.

A victim of violence may have the right to financial compensation from a government-funded scheme. A claim is made to the Criminal Injuries Compensation Authority (www.justice.gov.uk/victims-and-witnesses/cica), which is a government organisation that can pay compensation to people who have been physically or mentally injured because they were the blameless victim of a violent crime. It offers a free service, processing applications and making awards that range from £1000 to £500000.

Pursuing criminal proceedings

Each case must be considered on its merits, taking into account all available information about any mental health problem and its relevance to the offence, in addition to the principles set out in the *Code for Crown Prosecutors* (Crown Prosecution Service, 2010*a,b*). The *Code* explains that there is a balance to be struck between the public interest in diverting a defendant with significant mental illness from the criminal justice system and other public interest factors in favour of prosecution including the need to safeguard the public. If there is significant evidence to establish that a defendant or suspect has a significant mental illness, a prosecution may not be appropriate unless the offence is serious or there is a real possibility that it may be repeated, although some commentators have advocated for the reporting of all acts of non-trivial violence to the police (Wilson *et al*, 2012).

Chapter 11 discusses liaison with the police and the Crown Prosecution Service in more detail.

References

Bonner, G. & Wellman, N. (2010) Post-incident review of aggression and violence in mental health settings. *Journal of Psychosocial Nursing and Mental Health Services*, **48**, 35–40.

Crown Prosecution Service (2010*a*) *The Code for Crown Prosecutors*. CPS.

Crown Prosecution Service (2010*b*) Mentally disordered offenders. CPS (http://www.cps.gov.uk/legal/l_to_o/mentally_disordered_offenders/).

Kenardy, J. (2000) The current status of psychological debriefing. *BMJ*, **321**, 1032–1033.

McIvor, R. J., Canterbury, R. & Gunn, J. (1997) Psychological care of staff following traumatic incidents at work. *Psychiatric Bulletin*, **21**, 176–178.

National Institute for Mental Health in England (2004) *Developing Positive Practice to Support the Safe and Therapeutic Management of Aggression and Violence in Mental Health In-patient Settings*. Department of Health.

Raphael, B., Meldrum, L. & McFarlane, A. C. (1985) Does debriefing after psychological trauma work? Time for randomized controlled trials. *BMJ*, **310**, 1479–1480.

Rose, S. C., Bisson, J., Churchill, R., *et al* (2009) *Psychological Debriefing for Preventing Post Traumatic Stress Disorder (PTSD) (Review)*. Wiley.

Wilson, S., Murray, K., Harris, M., *et al* (2012) Psychiatric in-patients, violence and the criminal justice system. *The Psychiatrist*, **36**, 41–44.

Wykes, T. (1994) *Violence and Health Care Workers*. Chapman & Hall.

CHAPTER 7

Management of risk of violence in the community

James McIntyre, Elliot Wylde and Laura Garrod

Over the past 30 years, with the advent of community care, the establishment of functional community mental health teams and the use of SCT, psychiatric care is increasingly delivered in the community setting, often to patients who are acutely unwell and who in the past would have been treated on an in-patient unit. Furthermore, the management of violence in community settings is often problematic for a variety of reasons: the patient may be unknown to services, a response team may not be available, or the environment in which an assessment may take place may be unsuitable to manage the risk of violence.

Guidance on the psychiatric care of potentially violent patients in the community was provided by the Royal College of Psychiatrists in 2000. Its recommendations on the use of the care programme approach and risk management are now routine practice. The care programme approach provided mental health teams with a means to organise and record multi-agency working in a standardised manner. The report emphasised accurate, simple and quick systems for information transfer when a patient's care is moved between teams, including clarity with GPs on the responsibility for prescribing. In parallel with processes for efficient multidisciplinary working, it identified risk as an essential aspect of each patient's assessment. It also defined minimum requirements for risk assessment, recommended a multidisciplinary, structured approach, flexible to change, and the need for staff training to support this.

The Royal College of Psychiatrists' 2006 report on safety for psychiatrists defined the responsibilities of employing organisations such as NHS trusts for the safety of mental health professionals. These included statutory expectations with regard to policy, training and environment. The requirements included the need for trusts to develop policies on risk assessment in the community, reporting of untoward incidents, and on lone working. It highlighted the additional need for procedures to be put in place for support by other staff in emergencies and protocols for working with outside agencies such as the police. Staff training that was considered essential included breakaway, de-escalation, and risk assessment and management. Also necessary was regular review of safety measures such as clear exit facilities and adequate, functioning alarm systems.

This chapter reviews factors associated with violence in people with severe mental illness on which a community team may have a positive impact. It then looks at the common community situations in which safety needs particular consideration: on community visits, particularly when lone working, in out-patient clinics, and during Mental Health Act assessments in a private residence.

Modifiable factors associated with violence in the community

The risk of violence perpetrated by people with schizophrenia is low (Brennan *et al*, 2000; Fazel *et al*, 2009). However, there appears to be a subgroup representing less than 10–15% of those with mental illness that is responsible for the majority of violent acts (Steinert *et al*, 1998; Gje *et al*, 2003; Mullen, 2006). These individuals have several mediators of violence in addition to their mental illness. These factors interact, one increasing the likelihood that another will occur (Mullen, 2006; Volavka & Citrome, 2011).

These individuals are often male with a history of antisocial and/or violent behaviour or conduct disorder, a chaotic unstructured lifestyle, a history of substance misuse and consequently a disorganised clinical syndrome. In addition, these patients are less likely to be concordant with medication on discharge from hospital, more likely to disengage or be rejected by mental health and social support services, have experienced educational failure and unemployment, and have developed criminogenic peer groups.

There appears to be significant overlap of characteristics between this group and a part of the population identified in social studies as having severe multiple disadvantage. Individuals with severe multiple disadvantage have been shown to be particularly at risk of 'falling between the gaps' in the services society provides, while at the same time having among the most complex needs. Recommendations for social support in this group include more proactive outreach, individualised case management supporting client choice and user involvement, and multidisciplinary team working. The use of link-workers to support the formation of effective relationships between service users and key professionals, and to help them negotiate bureaucracy, has been shown to be a particularly useful and cost-effective intervention (Duncan & Corner, 2012).

From the mental health perspective these individuals may benefit from allocation of additional resources to ameliorate their risk. A structured multifactorial approach aiming for small improvements in a range of factors should be worthwhile, and is realistic in practice as often none will be entirely remedial. Areas in which a community team may be able to assist include (Mullen, 2006; Volavka, 2011):

- illness
- social context
- alcohol and substance misuse and comorbid mental disorder
- personality vulnerability.

Illness

Non-adherence to antipsychotic medication increases the risk of violence in schizophrenia (Ascher-Svanum *et al*, 2006) and is common (Lieberman *et al*, 2005). Although medication concordance can be closely monitored in in-patient settings, this is only possible with intensive support or with depot medication in the community. Decision-making regarding choice of medication is complicated, but the importance of adherence should be a higher priority where violence is more likely or historically more serious.

The strongest predictor for future non-adherence is non-adherence in the previous 6 months. Other indicators include recent illicit drug or alcohol use, prior treatment with an antidepressant, patient-reported medication-related cognitive impairment, history of violent behaviour and incarceration (Ascher-Svanum *et al*, 2006). In addition, hostility (Lindenmayer *et al*, 2009) and lack of insight (Mohammed *et al*, 2009) have been shown to predict non-concordance. Insight also predicts severity of violence in a concordant population, those with insight having better outcomes, and therefore insight appears to have an impact on propensity to violence by two independent pathways (Alia-Klein *et al*, 2007).

This suggests that when unsupervised oral medication is considered, persistence will be most likely in previously concordant individuals, with full resolution of symptoms, good insight and fewer side-effects (particularly cognitive). The greatest persistence in oral antipsychotic treatment was found for olanzapine in the European First Episode Schizophrenia Trial (EUFEST) (Kahn *et al*, 2008) and for clozapine in observational studies (Cooper *et al*, 2007). These studies may also suggest a role for eliciting and treating depressive symptoms where present and insight-oriented psychological work. There is no good evidence that high-dose antipsychotic prescribing is effective in chronic assaultive behaviour (Davison, 2005), rather that more side-effects lead to reduced adherence.

Where poor treatment adherence is likely or where relapse would be associated with a high potential risk, depot medication should be considered. A meta-analysis demonstrated that depot medications were superior to oral medications in preventing relapse (Leucht *et al*, 2011). Other work has indicated a reduction in rehospitalisation and discontinuation when oral and depot comparator preparations of the same drug were analysed (Tiihonen *et al*, 2011).

The evidence tends to suggest that treatment adherence and relapse rates may be improved by the use of depot antipsychotic medication even in the absence of SCT or other incentives. Depot medication also excludes the possibility of covert non-adherence.

Social context

It is true that SCT may facilitate adherence if other efforts have failed, however, its use also has the potential to damage the therapeutic alliance between a patient and their mental health team. The use of SCT should therefore not be considered an end in itself, but needs to be balanced with incentives that a patient values. A recovery approach that collaboratively supports a patient to develop their own hopes and goals and provides support to develop these is relevant, as it emphasises personal choice. In addition, balancing met need with patient responsibility encourages an adult–adult relationship to develop.

Input that patients may value include regular professional support, assistance developing structure in their lives, help to negotiate bureaucracy to gain benefits they are entitled to, and support developing new social networks, work-related skills and leisure activities (Mullen, 2006). Reoffending is also reduced by employment, stable relationships and by mixing with non-criminal peers.

Assistance to move to better accommodation is also valued by service users. People with schizophrenia tend to live in neighbourhoods characterised by high levels of disorder, fear of crime and victimisation. However, living in a socially disorganised neighbourhood increases the probability of violence in people with major mental illness (Silver, 2000). Where possible, high-risk patients are best served by placement in stable accommodation in low crime neighbourhoods.

Alcohol and substance misuse and comorbid mental disorder

Alcohol and substance misuse problems are common among patients in mental health services.

Use of alcohol and illicit drugs increases the risk of aggressive behaviour, particularly in psychotic conditions such as schizophrenia. Furthermore, psychotic illness is itself associated with a higher rate of comorbid substance misuse in comparison with the general population. Almost half of people with schizophrenia or schizophreniform disorder will receive a substance misuse diagnosis at some stage (OR = 4.6) (Volavka, 2011).

Violence may arise from the effects of the illicit drug use, from interaction between a mental illness and drug use, from illegal activities related to funding drug habits and by exposure to the sometimes violent illicit drug subculture of other drug users, drug dealers and gangs.

The assessment of patients with substance misuse and mental disorder should include a robust substance misuse history and enquiry about violence, particularly domestic violence. Monitoring (although difficult in practice) and management of substance misuse should be an important part of care planning. Approaches that take into consideration a service user's stage of change and consider harm minimisation as a viable goal are realistic and minimise the risk that community teams abandon this as a worthwhile area on which to focus their time and resources. Simply advising patients to stop taking illicit substances or alcohol does not work. Motivational interviewing as well as more active attempts to encourage treatment for substance misuse or dependence, including – if necessary – referral to drug or alcohol services, should form a component of routine clinical practice for patients with comorbid substance misuse and mental disorder (Royal College of Psychiatrists, 2008).

Personality vulnerability

Although active treatment of psychosis reduces the overall risk of violence in schizophrenia, analysis of CATIE (Clinical Antipsychotic Trials of Intervention Effectiveness) data has shown that adherence to antipsychotic medication did not significantly reduce incidents of violence in patients with a childhood antisocial history. This finding is consistent with the view that much of the violence in this group was related to underlying personality rather than psychosis and not likely to be improved by antipsychotic medication (Swanson *et al*, 2008).

There has been only limited success in the psychological treatment of severe personality disorder *per se*, however, individual personality elements are more modifiable. These include interpersonal skills training, anger control, effective self-assertion, victim empathy and the treatment of underlying cognitive distortions that underpin aggressive behaviour (Mullen, 2006). In addition, long-term psychosocial interventions using cognitive–behavioural approaches have been effective in reducing persistent aggressive behaviour in patients who are psychotic, although these programmes are expensive (Volavka, 2011).

Prosecution, although not feasible or desirable in all episodes of violence, may in some circumstances be of value to change the patient's legal status in a clinically helpful way, aid future risk assessment if offences are officially on record, and also to enable some patients to start taking responsibility for their actions (Davison, 2005).

Personal safety and lone working in the community

Trusts have an obligation under the Health and Safety at Work etc Act 1974 to provide a safe and secure environment for every member of staff. Procedures for maintaining safety when visiting patients in the community are now often set out in trust lone-working policies. Documents pertinent to lone working include *Not Alone* (NHS Security Management Service, 2005), *Tackling Violence Against Staff* (NHS Security Management Service, 2003) and *You're Not Alone* (Royal College of Nursing, 2007).

General considerations

Department managers should ensure that all staff working in the community or in isolated areas are trained and competent in interpersonal de-escalation, conflict resolution and breakaway skills. Ideally, training should be part of an induction period prior to starting employment, or as soon as possible afterwards, with annual refresher training made available.

When working in the community each staff member should consider their experience and limitations, including their health. This should include immunisation for tetanus, tuberculosis, hepatitis B and influenza. A clinician who is pregnant or who has a disability should carefully consider their potential vulnerability when visiting a patient's home. A professional appearance and a means of identification are appropriate and engender confidence. Flamboyant or sexually provocative clothing and expensive watches or jewellery should not be worn in case they are provocative to a patient. Similarly, items that could potentially be used to strangle or injure such as necklaces, scarves or fountain pens are best avoided.

Prior to a visit, a risk assessment is necessary in order to identify whether it is appropriate to go alone or with support. Staff should gain information about the patient, their family and the local environment prior to the visit. This may include the visit address, forensic history, substance misuse, carers and pets. The police may be able to provide information when concern is raised regarding risk of violence.

In general, initial visits should be in pairs unless there is clear evidence of low risk (e.g. in older persons' services if seeing someone with memory impairment (Royal College of Psychiatrists, 2006)). Similarly, out-of-hours visits should always be conducted by two people. The workers should meet at a pre-arranged place before the visit (e.g. the local hospital or in a public place) and travel together to the visit from there. Meeting at the patient's home or in the street should be avoided if at all possible. If an individual is assessed as high risk, consider whether the police should also attend, or if in a public place consider whether it may be more appropriate to ask the police to detain the patient and take them to a place of safety, where the assessment can take place. If the patient is considered low risk, visiting alone is reasonable (Galloway, 2002).

It is good practice to inform families of a visit and the approximate arrival time, although clinical judgement is necessary with regard to informing the patient. Consider also whether an interpreter will be necessary. Once you have arrived at a patient's home, staff should stand back from the door after ringing the bell. Be prepared to abort the visit if the patient refuses to be seen, is intoxicated with drugs or alcohol, or is not alone, until adequate safeguards can be put in place. If the visit proceeds, the occupants should be followed into the residence, making a mental note of the environment and potential escape routes. If the patient has a dog, it is wise to ask for it to be kept in another room.

It is worthwhile to consider whether the assessment is feasible and/or desirable if a family member is present. In some situations, for example where there is concern regarding domestic violence or where a person may be reticent to disclose symptoms in front of family members, it may be preferable to interview the patient and family separately. At the same time, cultural factors such as the gender of the staff member and an expectation of family presence should be respected. Give plenty of personal space and ideally try to place oneself between the patient and the exit door.

When first meeting a patient, introduce oneself and produce identification. It is also advisable to ask how the patient would like to be addressed. If note-taking it is polite to ask the patient whether they mind and avoid taking notes if they are suspicious. Communicate clearly about the task, and be sensitive to personal dignity (particularly if neighbours are aware of the visit). The patient should be given the opportunity to terminate the interview if at any time they feel too uncomfortable, and the staff member should also be prepared to close the interview if they feel threatened.

If blocked from leaving, contact the team base, maintain an adequate distance, and explain your intentions to the patient and to others present. Move towards the door and avoid corners. If a weapon is produced, ask for it to be put down rather than handed over. Try to appear calm, and ensure verbal and non-verbal communication is non-threatening. A solution-focused approach encouraging collaboration is a helpful de-escalation tool; therefore engage in conversation, acknowledge concerns and feelings, and ask for facts about the patient's problems (Galloway, 2002; Royal College of Psychiatrists, 2006).

Specific considerations when lone working

Local protocols for lone working

Local protocols for lone working should include arrangements for:

- signing in and out of buildings
- tracking staff whereabouts and reporting off duty at the end of the shift/working day
- registering car identification details
- maintaining regular contact with staff who work alone in the community
- ensuring community staff carry a work mobile telephone and that in-patient staff carry one with them when leaving the hospital on escort duty.

Staff should be aware of team procedures for keeping in touch with base, and action to be taken in an emergency. Base should know where their staff are at all times, and should be informed of any change in itinerary. A white board in the main office detailing planned visits of all staff and indicating whether they are currently in or out of the office is one way the team can know where staff should be. Alternatively, diary details of visits can be left at a central point. Staff must leave detailed particulars of where they are going and a definite time by which they will return or make contact. A contingency plan should be in place if that staff member does not return or make contact at the agreed time. Staff should ensure that they return at the expected time or contact the office to say they are delayed unless an emergency arises. If a worker fails to return, every effort should be made to ascertain where they are. The manager or designated deputy will be informed. Continued failure to identify the whereabouts of the staff member will result in them being reported as a missing person to the police. It can also be a useful safety check for staff to telephone base at the end of the day when their visits are completed.

High-risk visits

Members of staff should never visit alone or if awaiting other agencies enter a building alone on such visits. High-risk visits include visits to:

- unknown individuals threatening violence
- unknown individuals where no risk assessment has been carried out
- known individuals with a history of serious violence, now refusing to engage with the service
- known individuals with no history of violence, but who are now unwell and threatening violence
- individuals who have been reported as being actively suicidal or at risk of self-harm
- individuals who are known to be intoxicated with drugs, alcohol or other substances, increasing the risk of violence or self-harm
- individuals who live with others with a history of violence or drug/ alcohol misuse
- areas or housing estates where it is not considered safe to visit alone, especially after dark.

When planning such a visit consider whether it is possible to see the person at the team base or other community centre where back-up is available. Police presence may be required if there is a risk of violence. Each team must agree local arrangements with the police for situations where help may be required. A visit should not go ahead until police assistance has been secured if staff members are concerned about safety. Police may request a risk assessment in advance in these circumstances.

Safety in the out-patient setting

If members of the community team are using community facilities it is the trust's responsibility to ensure that the safety standards for a psychiatric interview room are met (Royal College of Psychiatrists, 1999; Galloway, 2002; Davison, 2005). These include:

- easily accessible, functioning alarm systems, with a protocol for responding
- clear, unobstructed exits
- an exit that is safe: doors that open outward, cannot be locked from the inside and allow easy access from the outside in the event of an emergency
- location close to staff areas
- removal of all potential weapons such as paperweights

- an unobstructed viewing window
- a furniture layout that minimises the potential for violence, with the staff member and patient having equal access to the door, neither barred from exiting by the other.

In addition to environmental factors, a number of procedures are also recommended in order to maintain safety in the out-patient setting (NHS Employers, 2011).

- Reception staff should be appropriately protected and never isolated.
- Staff should not work alone in isolated rooms if this can be avoided.
- Staff should be aware of their colleagues' whereabouts.
- As far as possible, one person is not opening or locking premises alone in darkness, particularly if drugs or other target items are kept on the premises.
- Staff must not arrange to see a patient after 17.00 h at the office base without assessing risk and arranging colleague cover at the time. If a member of staff were to find themself alone in a building with a patient, they should cancel the appointment.
- Staff should be discouraged from working alone at their base after hours and should be aware of the possible risks involved. If this cannot be avoided there must be protocols in place to minimise risks such as the staff member informing an identified member of the team that they are working late, stating expected finish time and contacting the team member to inform them when they have safely left the building.

When seeing a patient, recognition that the out-patient interview can be very stressful can do much to alleviate anxiety and the potential for agitated behaviour. If the patient has been waiting for some time beyond the agreed appointment time, it is appropriate to offer an apology. If a patient appears highly aroused or under the influence of drugs or alcohol it is reasonable to consider whether the interview should be postponed, and if the interview is to continue it is preferable that a colleague also attends.

Standards of safety may be lower in community facilities that are shared with specialties facing a lower degree of risk, such as GP surgeries. If minimum safety standards are not in place this should be reported to the trust management. In the meantime, temporary safety precautions can be implemented: ensure someone is within hearing distance; if the room is isolated, request a member of the clinic staff to be available outside the room; use a personal alarm if no permanent alarm is installed and inform the clinic staff of its meaning if it is set off. Finally, rearrange the furniture as appropriate.

Mental Health Act assessments

Mental Health Act assessments can be emotionally charged affairs and are often stressful for the patient, carers and the professionals involved.

Thorough preparation and effective communication are the key to safe management, and guidance is given here regarding best practice in this area (London Development Centre for Mental Health, 2005).

Planned assessments

Mental Health Act assessments of persons on private property are carried out by an approved mental health professional (AMHP), Section 12-approved doctors and doctors with prior knowledge of the patient (e.g. their GP). The assessment is arranged and controlled by the AMHP who holds ultimate responsibility for the management of the assessment.

Before carrying out a mental health assessment the AMHP has the responsibility of gathering relevant background information in order to undertake a risk assessment on a person in accordance with the local authority's risk management procedures. This will enable the AMHP to determine how the assessment can be safely implemented and whether police presence is required. Risks to be assessed will include:

- the potential for violence to self and others
- the potential for self-harm
- resistance to entry for purposes of assessment
- resistance to removal to hospital once an assessment has been completed.

The information gathered for this purpose will include information from:

- the referrer
- next of kin, family member or carer
- existing risk assessment documentation, care plan, contingency and crisis plans
- the police, if the patient is thought to have a significant criminal record
- other sources where appropriate (e.g. friend, neighbour, housing association).

The AMHP should also carefully assess whether there are issues pertaining to language or other potential communication problems, disability, race, ethnicity, sexuality or gender that may require special consideration. If children are involved, the AMHP may, where appropriate, consider contacting the child and family service.

The outcome of the information-gathering will influence the decision whether to request police attendance at the assessment. If it is deemed necessary then the AMHP will liaise directly with the police. Currently there remains a degree of difference in protocols agreed between various police forces and mental health trusts. Many now have agreed that when police involvement is requested, the AMHP will complete a police risk assessment form and fax/email this to the police. The police should receive as much advance notice as practicable of the need for their assistance.

On contacting the police, the AMHP should speak to the duty controller and provide the following information:

- time and address of the proposed assessment
- name and date of birth of the person to be assessed
- the reason for police involvement in the assessment
- contact details of the AMHP responsible for the assessment process
- details of any other person likely to be on the premises
- details of any history of violence
- any other known or potential risks.

On receipt of this information the police will create an intelligence record, conduct a risk assessment ensuring that searches of criminal intelligence databases are carried out, and consider any other police-held information which may need to be disclosed to the AMHP prior to attending the address. It is the responsibility of the police to determine the level of response required, and the responsibility of the operations office inspector to ensure appropriate resources are identified, tasked and briefed.

Where several agencies are involved in the assessment (e.g. police, local ambulance service, mental health staff), it is good practice immediately before the assessment to discuss any risk issues, roles and responsibilities and to agree an action plan, having given consideration to all possible circumstances, including who has control of the scene both generally and if specific scenarios occur.

If, following the assessment, the decision is made to detain the person, then the Mental Health Act allows for the removal of that person from the premises on which they have been assessed, in order to be admitted to hospital. It is the AMHP's responsibility to ensure that the patient's admission to hospital is carried out in a safe and humane way.

The way in which the decision is conveyed to the patient can make all the difference. If the patient is receptive, it might be helpful to explain in clear language exactly what has been decided. If the patient is not known to psychiatric services, it might also be helpful to explain what to expect from a hospital admission, where it will take place, how long the assessment and possible treatment will take, and visiting arrangements for the family. These phrases can be helpful:

- 'We do understand that we may not be in agreement about this, but we have decided that you need a period in hospital for your own health'
- 'We do think that on the basis of our discussions it is important to assess whether you have mental health problems, and the safest place to carry this out is in hospital'
- 'We can assure you that we will not keep you in hospital any longer than is necessary in order to make sure that everything is alright'.

It is the responsibility of the police to prevent any breach of the peace and to protect people and property. Section 137 of the Mental Health Act gives power to any police constable, the AMHP or conveying personnel (e.g. ambulance crew) to use force to detain a person who has been assessed under the Mental Health Act, who is in need of admission to hospital but who resists, or where there is considered to be a significant risk of violence. However, police transport should only be used to convey the person to hospital if they are violent or potentially violent, or where they may be a danger to the public.

If police transport is used, the detained person should, wherever possible, be accompanied by a member of the ambulance crew who can monitor the person's mental and physical condition, with the ambulance following. This may not always be possible, and the person should be conveyed to hospital as quickly as possible, avoiding any delay that could lead to increased risk or distress for the patient and others.

Assessments in the community without police in attendance

During the initial information-gathering phase, the AMHP in conjunction with other members of the multidisciplinary team may have concluded that police presence was not necessary. However, they should still consider in advance:

- what action they will take if they are met at the scene by violence or resistance
- what action they will take if the person being assessed passively resists once the papers are completed.

There should also be a robust process in place by which an AMHP can urgently enlist the help of the police (e.g. through the borough control room or operations or events office). Arrangements for out-of-hours requests should also be in place.

When a pre-planned assessment has been conducted without police involvement, but because of threatening behaviour or violence displayed during the assessment it becomes necessary to call police for assistance, use should be made of the 999 emergency system. In such cases the AMHP should contact the police control room and request urgent assistance. The duty officer will then assume responsibility for dealing with the request for assistance and ensuring a satisfactory conclusion.

Debriefing

Once the person has been assessed and either safely conveyed to hospital or the decision made to offer alternative treatment, a debriefing should take place between the AMHP and the police attending the scene in order to discuss any problems or suggestions arising. Other multidisciplinary team members present during the assessment need not always be available for the debriefing and it remains the responsibility of the AMHP to ensure all parties are satisfied with the decision-making process and have had the opportunity to feedback any suggestions or concerns.

References

Alia-Klein, N., O'Rourke, T. M., Goldstein, R. Z., et al (2007) Insight into illness and adherence to psychotropic medications are separately associated with violence severity in a forensic sample. *Aggressive Behaviour*, **33**, 86–96.

Ascher-Svanum, H., Zhu, B., Faries, D., et al (2006) Prospective study of risk factors for non adherence with antipsychotic medication in the treatment of schizophrenia. *Journal of Clinical Psychiatry*, **67**, 1114–1123.

Brennan, P. A., Mednick, S. A. & Hodgins, S. (2000) Major mental disorders and criminal violence in a Danish birth cohort. *Archives of General Psychiatry*, **57**, 494–500.

Cooper, D., Moisan, J. & Gregoire, J. P. (2007) Adherence to atypical antipsychotic treatment among newly treated patients: a population based study in schizophrenia. *Journal of Clinical Psychiatry*, **68**, 818–825.

Davison, S. E. (2005) The management of violence in general psychiatry. *Advances in Psychiatric Treatment*, **11**, 362–370.

Duncan, M. & Corner, J. (2012) *Severe and Multiple Disadvantage: A Review of Key Texts*. Lankelly Chase Foundation.

Fazel, S., Gulati, G., Linsell, L., et al (2009) Schizophrenia and violence: systematic review and meta-analysis. *PLoS Medicine*, **6**, e1000120.

Galloway, J. (2002) Personal safety when visiting patients in the community. *Advances in Psychiatric Treatment*, **8**, 214–222.

Gje, X., Brent Donnellan, M. & Wenk, E. (2003) Differences in personality and patterns of recidivism between early starters and other serious male offenders. *Journal of the American Academy of Psychiatry and the Law*, **31**, 68–77.

Kahn, R. S., Fleischenhacker, W. W., Boter, H., et al (2008) Effectiveness of antipsychotic drugs in first episode schizophrenia and schizophreniform disorder: an open randomized clinical trial. *Lancet*, **371**, 1085–1097.

Leucht, C., Heres, S., Kane, J. M., et al (2011) Oral versus depot antipsychotics for schizophrenia – a critical systematic review and meta-analysis of randomized long term trials. *Schizophrenia Research*, **127**, 83–92.

Lieberman, J. A., Stroup, T. S., McEvoy, J. P., et al (2005) Effectiveness of antipsychotic drugs in patients with schizophrenia. *New England Journal of Medicine*, **353**, 1209–1223.

Lindenmayer, J. P., Liu-Seifert, H., Kulkarni, P. M., et al (2009) Medication non adherence and treatment outcome in patients with schizophrenia and schizoaffective disorder with suboptimal prior response. *Journal of Clinical Psychiatry*, **70**, 990–996.

London Development Centre for Mental Health (2005) *Joint Protocol for Assesments on Private Premises (Section 135 Mental Health Act 1983)*. Barnet, Enfield and Haringey Mental Health NHS Trust.

Mohammed, S., Rosenheck, R., McEvoy, J., et al (2009) Cross sectional and longitudinal relationships between insight and attitudes toward medication and clinical outcomes in chronic schizophrenia. *Schizophrenia Bulletin*, **35**, 336–346.

Mullen, P. E. (2006) Schizophrenia and violence: from correlations to preventive strategies. *Advances in Psychiatric Treatment*, **12**, 239–248.

NHS Employers (2011) *Lone Working*. NHS Employers (http://www.nhsemployers.org/Aboutus/Publications/Documents/Lone%20working.pdf).

NHS Security Management Service (2003) *Tackling Violence Against Staff*. NHS Security Management Service.

NHS Security Management Service (2005) *Not Alone: A Good Practice Guide for the Better Protection of Lone Workers in the NHS*. NHS Security Management Service.

Royal College of Nursing (2007) *You're Not Alone. The RCN – Campaigning to Protect Lone Workers*. Royal College of Nursing.

Royal College of Psychiatrists (1999) *Safety for Trainees in Psychiatry: Report of the Collegiate Trainees' Committee Working Party on the Safety of Trainees* (Council Report CR78). Royal College of Psychiatrists.

Royal College of Psychiatrists (2000) *Good Medical Practice in the Psychiatric Care of Potentially Violent Patients in the Community* (Council Report CR80). Royal College of Psychiatrists.

Royal College of Psychiatrists (2006) *Safety for Psychiatrists* (Council Report CR134). Royal College of Psychiatrists.

Royal College of Psychiatrists (2008) *Rethinking Risk to Others in Mental Health Services* (College Report CR150). Royal College of Psychiatrists.

Silver, E. (2000) Extending social disorganisation theory: a multilevel approach to the study of violence among persons with mental illness. *Criminology*, **38**, 1043–1074.

Steinert, T., Darjee, R. & Thompson, L. D. G. (1998) Violence and schizophrenia: two types of criminal offenders. *European Journal of Psychiatry*, **12**, 153–165.

Swanson, J. W., Swartz, M. S., Van Dorn, R. A., *et al* (2008) Comparison of antipsychotic medication effects on reducing violence in people with schizophrenia. *British Journal of Psychiatry*, **193**, 37–43.

Tiihonen, J., Haukka, J., Taylor, M., *et al* (2011) A nationwide cohort study of oral and depot antipsychotics after first hospitalization for schizophrenia. *American Journal of Psychiatry*, **168**, 603–609.

Volavka, J. (2011) Schizophrenia, treatment adherence, substance use, and violence. In *Proceedings of the 7th European Congress on Violence in Clinical Psychiatry* (eds I. Needham, H. Nijman, T. Palmstierna, *et al*), pp. 42–49. Kavanah.

Volavka, J. & Citrome, L. (2011) Pathways to aggression in schizophrenia affect results of treatment. *Schizophrenia Bulletin*, **37**, 921–929.

CHAPTER 8

Management of violence in older adults

Jonathan Waite

How big is the problem?

Nearly 700 000 people in the UK are thought to have dementia (Knapp & Prince, 2007), making this by far the most prevalent serious mental disorder. Approximately 90% will develop behavioural or psychological symptoms as a result of their dementia, and in about 13% the predominant problem will be physical aggression (Waite *et al*, 2008: p. 153). Functional psychiatric illnesses may continue with ageing or present for the first time in older adults, but this chapter will concentrate on the management of violence in older people with organic disorders.

The Healthcare Commission's *National Audit of Violence 2006–2007* (Healthcare Commission, 2008*a,b*) included for the first time incidents of violence in hospital services for older people, in addition to those occurring in units for adults of working age. The findings were disturbing but not widely publicised. It appears from the accounts of service users and carers that the quality of nursing being delivered in the hospital wards studied was extremely high, but this was not enough to prevent physical violence being a distressingly frequent event.

- Nurses working in older people's services were more likely to have experienced physical assault (64% had been assaulted) than those employed in services for adults of working age.
- In older people's services, violent incidents were less likely to be precipitated by too rapid use of medication or physical restraint.
- Older people's wards were less well designed and equipped, with poorer sightlines, poorer control of heating and ventilation, and less easy access to resuscitation equipment.
- Alarm systems and training were less satisfactory in older people's units.
- Nursing staff had less influence on admission policy and more difficulties in accessing additional staff in older people's units.

About 500 000 people live in care homes in the UK. Data on care home populations are not routinely collected in the UK, but in Scotland about

90% of care home places (38341/42810) are for elderly people (Information Services Division, 2011). Even in homes not specifically registered to provide care for people with mental disorder, the majority of residents have dementia – about 80% of residents of non-specialist homes are thought to have dementia (Knapp & Prince, 2007) – compared with nearly 90% of those in designated specialist EMI (elderly mentally infirm) units. The main function of long-stay care for older people is now to provide care to people with dementia (MacDonald & Cooper, 2007). Challenging behaviours exhibited towards family and other informal carers are an important factor in people with dementia being placed in care homes (Donaldson et al, 1997).

Much attention has been given to abuse of residents by staff in care homes, but the complementary issue of abuse of care staff by residents is not generally acknowledged (Zeller et al, 2009). There are no reliable recent data on the prevalence of violent episodes in UK care homes, but it is likely that the situation is more serious in care homes in the community. From the limited audits that have been conducted, one staff survey (Goodridge et al, 1996) found that 85% of staff reported being psychologically abused in the past month, and 60% had been physically assaulted. Staff could expect on average to be insulted 11.3 times each month and assaulted 9.3 times each month. Another study (Hagen & Sayers, 1995) found that in a 200-bedded care home observed over 8 days, there were 182 acts of physical aggression directed against staff, resulting in 11 significant injuries.

What is the current guidance?

Many organisations have produced guidance on the management of challenging behaviour in older people, mostly concentrating on individuals with dementia (Royal College of Nursing, 2004; National Institute for Health and Clinical Excellence & Social Care Institute for Excellence, 2006; Scottish Intercollegiate Guideline Network, 2006; Commission for Social Care Inspection, 2007a,b; National Collaborating Centre for Mental Health, 2007), emphasising the importance of skilled nursing and adopting the principles of person-centred care. Full accounts of the practice of person-centred care can be found in Brooker (2008) and Waite et al (2008).

The NICE dementia guideline (2006) acknowledges that mediation will sometimes be required and repeats the advice given in other NICE publications on techniques of drug administration and monitoring. The advice is contradictory: paragraph 1.7.3.6 states that 'violent behaviour should be managed without the prescription of high doses or combinations of drugs', but paragraph 1.7.3.13. states that 'if rapid tranquillisation is needed a combination of IM [intramuscular] haloperidol and IM lorazepam should be considered'. The guidance is otherwise in agreement with the recommendations in Chapter 6 (p. 55).

A key driver has been the concern that older people in care homes have been indiscriminately prescribed medication (Banerjee, 2009). In response to Banerjee's report, the Alzheimer's Society (2011) and the Royal College of Nursing (Sturdy, 2012) have produced good practice guidance on reducing the use of antipsychotics.

The British Geriatrics Society & College of Emergency Medicine (2012) have produced guidance (endorsed by many professional bodies) on the management of older people in emergency departments.

The running of registered care homes is controlled by the Care Standards Act 2000 supplemented by the Care Homes Regulations 2001 (Department of Health, 2003). Inspection and registration of homes is undertaken by the Care Quality Commission. The duty to comply with legal procedures is placed on the registered person who runs the home. Among other duties, the registered person must:

- ensure that the care home is conducted so as to promote and make proper provision for the health and welfare of service users
- enable service users to make decisions with respect to the care they are to receive and their health and welfare
- ascertain and take into account service users' wishes and feelings
- conduct the home in a manner which respects the privacy and dignity of service users
- ensure that unnecessary risks to the health or safety of service users are identified and so far as possible eliminated
- make suitable arrangements to provide a safe system for moving and handling service users
- make the service user's plan available to the service user and keep the plan under review
- give notice to the Care Quality Commission without delay of any event which adversely affects the well-being or safety of any service user.

There are specific regulations with regard to physical restraint; no service user should be subject to physical restraint unless:

- restraint is the only practicable means of securing the welfare of that or any other service user and there are exceptional circumstances
- the restraint is allowed under Section 6 of the Mental Capacity Act 2005
- every time restraint is used, the circumstances – including the nature of the restraint – must be recorded.

Evidence

Despite its widespread advocacy there is surprisingly little evidence that person-centred care and other non-pharmacological therapies are effective in preventing aggression (Allen-Burge *et al*, 1999; Chenoweth *et al*, 2009), although it has been shown that enhanced psychosocial care can reduce the need for medication (Fossey *et al*, 2006).

Staff education can certainly help (Hagen & Sayers 1995; Zeller *et al* 2009), but as the Healthcare Commission (2008*b*) survey showed, even highly trained and experienced nurses can be the victims of serious violence.

Although there is limited evidence for the efficacy of antipsychotic medication in dementia, with little benefit being found in the reduction of agitation and psychosis, it has been a consistent finding that antipsychotic medication has a significant effect in reducing levels of aggression (Lonergan *et al*, 2002; Ballard *et al*, 2006). However, the effect size is modest, the duration of benefit may be brief and there are likely to be adverse effects if treatment is continued (Ballard *et al*, 2009).

Anticonvulsants have only been subjected to small-scale trials in older adults with challenging behaviour. A study of carbamazepine (Tariot *et al* 1998) showed some benefit but also troublesome adverse effects; hopes from a pilot study that valproate might be effective and better tolerated were not confirmed in larger studies (Lonergan *et al*, 2009).

Trazodone has been widely used to treat agitation, although the largest study did not demonstrate significant benefit (Teri *et al*, 2000). Citalopram showed effects comparable to risperidone in one trial (Pollock *et al*, 2007), but Banerjee *et al* (2011) were unable to show benefit in depressive symptoms in patients with dementia treated with sertraline or mirtazepine.

Cholinesterase inhibitor drugs do not reduce and may even increase levels of agitation (Howard *et al*, 2007); adding sertraline makes little difference (Finkel *et al*, 2004). Memantine has become popular for the treatment of agitation in dementia despite absence of evidence from prospective controlled studies. There is no evidence that it is effective in acutely violent patients.

There is little evidence on rapid tranquillisation. Meehan *et al* (2002) found that intramuscular lorazepam (1 mg) and olanzapine (2.5–5.0 mg) were effective in reducing agitation and excitation, without producing sedation, cardiac conduction abnormalities or EPS. The reduction in excitation was more prolonged with olanzapine.

Practical management of potentially violent older people

The application of basic principles of person-centred care and behavioural management should minimise the risk of violence. If violence is a result of inappropriate care of the patient and it is not possible to expeditiously educate the carers, then it is usually best to try to arrange alternative placement where more sensitive care can be provided.

However, moving such patients can provoke more violence, even if the carers in the new environment are skilled and experienced. In these circumstances prophylactic use of sedation should be considered, following the guidelines in Chapter 5.

Environmental factors may provoke or exacerbate violence, for example:

- noise
- heat
- cold
- interference by other residents.

These factors may interact with poor hearing and eyesight to increase levels of suspicion and fear.

Apart from inappropriate care, the most likely cause of violence is physical discomfort, including:

- pain
- constipation
- breathlessness
- urinary retention
- incontinence.

Violence may be the first sign of physical illness – urinary tract infection is the most commonly considered condition but the presentation of disease in confused elderly people is notoriously non-specific. Sometimes the diagnosis becomes apparent on physical examination, but negative findings do not exclude the possibility of serious illness. There is a real dilemma in deciding the best environment in which to provide the most appropriate care. There are no hard and fast rules, but the factors in Table 8.1 should be considered.

Table 8.1 Facilities for the care of a potentially violent older person

Environment	Advantages	Disadvantages
Home	Familiarity Transport not required	Carers may lack training Back-up not readily available Limited facilities for investigation and diagnosis
Care home	May be familiar 24-hour care	Staff may lack skills Limited facilities for investigation and diagnosis Other residents may be distressed by violent disturbed patient
Acute hospital	Good facilities for diagnosis and treatment 24-hour care Ready access to back-up	Unfamiliar and possibly distressing environment Staff may lack understanding of mental disorders Other patients may be distressed by violent disturbed patient
Mental health unit	Staff experienced at management of disturbed behaviour Access to back-up	Staff may lack skill at managing physical illness Other patients may exacerbate disturbance

Recommendations

Banerjee (2009) concluded that:

- antipsychotics should not be a first-line treatment except in circumstances of extreme risk and harm;
- the first-line of management should be detailed assessment to identify any treatable cause of behavioural and psychological symptoms of dementia (e.g. delirium, pain, depression); this should include taking the history of the problem, having the behaviour described by the carer/team, and discussing current and past behaviour with the carer/team.

This is sound advice but it is important to remember that old people with disturbed behaviour often have physical disorders. To make a physical assessment and diagnosis, it is justified to resort to the use of medication to allow an adequate physical assessment if experienced medical and nursing staff are unable to de-escalate the situation causing violence. The prescription of tranquillising medication should be reviewed once the assessment has been completed and effective treatment has been initiated, but it is often prudent to continue until the patient is settled back in their home.

References

Allen-Burge, R., Stevens, A. B. & Burgio, L. D. (1999) Effective behavioural interventions for decreasing dementia-related challenging behaviour in nursing homes. *International Journal of Geriatric Psychiatry*, **14**, 213–228.

Alzheimer's Society (2011) *Reducing the Use of Antipsychotic Drugs: A Guide to the Treatment and Care of Behavioural and Psychological Symptoms of Dementia*. Alzheimer's Society.

Ballard, C. G., Birks, J. & Waite, J. (2006) Atypical antipsychotics for aggression and psychosis in Alzheimer disease. *Cochrane Database of Systematic Reviews*, **1**, CD003476.

Ballard, C. G., Hanney, M. L., Theodoulou, M., *et al* (2009) The dementia antipsychotic withdrawal trial (DART-AD): long-term follow-up of a randomised placebo-controlled trial. *Lancet Neurology*, **8**, 151–157.

Banerjee, S. (2009) *The Use of Antipsychotic Medication for People with Dementia: Time for Action*. Department of Health.

Banerjee, S., Hellier, J., Dewey, M., *et al* (2011) Sertraline or mirtazapine for depression in dementia (HTA-SADD): a randomised, multicentre, double-blind, placebo-controlled trial. *Lancet*, **378**, 403–411.

British Geriatrics Society & College of Emergency Medicine (2012) *The Silver Book: Quality Care for Older People with Urgent and Emergency Care Needs*. British Geriatrics Society.

Brooker, D. (2008) Person centred care. In *Oxford Textbook of Old Age Psychiatry* (eds R. Jacoby, C. Oppenheimer, T. Dening, *et al*), pp. 229–240. Oxford University Press.

Chenoweth, L., King, M. T., Jeon, Y. H., *et al* (2009) Caring for aged dementia care resident study (CADRES) of person-centred care, dementia care mapping and usual care in dementia: a cluster randomised trial. *Lancet Neurology*, **8**, 317–325.

Commission for Social Care Inspection (2007a) *Rights, Risks and Restraints: An Exploration into the Use of Restraint with Older People*. CSCI.

Commission for Social Care Inspection (2007b) *Guidance for Inspectors: How to Move Towards Restraint-free Care*. CSCI.

Department of Health (2003) *Care Homes for Older People: National Minimum Standards. Care Homes Regulations* (Third Edition). TSO (The Stationery Office).

Donaldson, C., Tarrier, N. & Burns, A. (1997) The impact of the symptoms of dementia on caregivers. *British Journal of Psychiatry*, **170**, 62–68.

Finkel, S. I., Mintzer, J. E., Dysken, M., *et al* (2004) A randomized, placebo-controlled study of the efficacy and safety of sertraline in the treatment of the behavioral manifestations of Alzheimer's disease in outpatients treated with donepezil. *International Journal of Geriatric Psychiatry*, **19**, 9–18.

Fossey, J., Ballard, C., Juszczak, E., *et al* (2006) Effect of enhanced psychosocial care on antipsychotic use in nursing home residents with severe dementia: cluster randomized trial. *BMJ*, **332**, 756.

Goodridge, D. M., Johnston, P. & Thompson, M. (1996) Conflict and aggression as stressors in the work environment of nursing assistants: implications for institutional elder abuse. *Journal of Elder Abuse and Neglect*, **8**, 49–67.

Hagen, B. F. & Sayers, D. (1995) When caring leaves bruises: the effects of staff education on resident aggression. *Journal of Gerontological Nursing*, **21**, 7–16.

Healthcare Commission (2008a) *National Audit of Violence 2006–7: Final Report – Working Age Adult Services*. Royal College of Psychiatrists' Centre for Quality Improvement.

Healthcare Commission (2008b) *National Audit of Violence 2006–7: Final Report – Older People's Services*. Royal College of Psychiatrists' Centre for Quality Improvement.

Howard, R. J., Juszczak, E., Ballard, C. G., *et al* (2007) Donepezil for the treatment of agitation in Alzheimer's disease. *New England Journal of Medicine*, **357**, 1382–1392.

Information Services Division (2011) *Care Home Census 2011 – Interim Analysis*. ISD, NHS National Services Scotland.

Knapp, M. & Prince, M. (2007) *Dementia UK: A Report into the Prevalence and Cost of Dementia*. Alzheimer's Society.

Lonergan, E., Luxenberg, J., Colford, J. M., *et al* (2002) Haloperidol for agitation in dementia. *Cochrane Database of Systematic Reviews*, **2**, CD002852.

Lonergan, E., Luxenberg, J., Colford, J. M., *et al* (2009) Valproate preparations for agitation in dementia. *Cochrane Database of Systematic Reviews*, **3**, CD003945.

MacDonald, A. & Cooper, B. (2007) Long-term care and dementia services: an impending crisis. *Age and Ageing*, **36**, 16–22.

Meehan, K. M., Wang, H., David, S. R., *et al* (2002) Comparison of rapidly acting intramuscular olanzapine, lorazepam and placebo: a double-blind randomized study in acutely agitated patients with dementia. *Neuropsychopharmacology*, **26**, 494–504.

National Collaborating Centre for Mental Health (2007) *Dementia: A NICE–SCIE Guideline on Supporting People with Dementia and Their Carers in Health and Social Care* (National Clinical Practice Guideline CG42). British Psychological Society & Gaskell.

National Institute for Health and Clinical Excellence & Social Care Institute for Excellence (2006) *Dementia: Supporting People with Dementia and Their Carers in Health and Social Care*. NICE.

Pollock, B. G., Mulsant, B. H., Rosen, J., *et al* (2007) A double-blind comparison of citalopram and risperidone for the treatment of behavioral and psychotic symptoms associated with dementia. *American Journal of Geriatric Psychiatry*, **15**, 942–952.

Royal College of Nursing (2004) *Restraint Revisited – Rights, Risk, Responsibility: Guidance for Nursing Staff*. RCN.

Scottish Intercollegiate Guidelines Network (2006) *Management of Patients with Dementia* (*Guideline 86*). SIGN.

Sturdy, D. (2012) *Antipsychotic Drugs in Dementia: A Best Practice Guide*. Royal College of Nursing & Nursing Standard.

Tariot, P. N., Erb, R., Podgorski, C. A., *et al* (1998) Efficacy and tolerability of carbamazepine for agitation and aggression in dementia. *American Journal of Psychiatry*, **155**, 54–61.

Teri, L., Logsdon, R. G., Peskind, E., *et al* (2000) Treatment of agitation in dementia: a randomized placebo controlled trial. *Neurology*, **55**, 1271–1278.

Waite, J., Harwood, R., Morton, I., *et al* (2008) *Dementia Care: A Practical Manual.* Oxford University Press.

Zeller, A., Hahn, S., Needham, I., *et al* (2009) Aggressive behavior of nursing home residents towards caregivers: a systematic literature review. *Geriatric Nursing,* **30,** 174–187.

CHAPTER 9

Management of violence in people with intellectual disability

Ingrid Bohnen, Alina Bakala, Yogesh Thakker
and Anusha Wijeratne

Violent behaviour displayed by individuals with intellectual disability is one of the biggest challenges to services. It is one of many manifestations of challenging behaviour. It may include punching, slapping, pushing, pulling, kicking, pinching, scratching, pulling hair, biting, head butting, using weapons, choking and throttling, and sexual violence. Violence can occur in a variety of settings: in in-patient and community-based settings such as family homes, settings run by statutory organisations as well as those in the private and voluntary sector. Children with intellectual disability and severe challenging aggressive behaviour may be placed in residential schools.

Violent behaviour has many serious consequences for both individuals with intellectual disability and formal and informal carers, and is a major obstacle to the individual's social integration. Violent behaviour is also one of the main reasons for referral to mental health professionals and services. Often violent behaviour leads to multiple admissions to institutions and psychiatric facilities. Staff working with individuals with intellectual disability who experience challenging behaviour, including violent behaviour, may experience high levels of stress and burnout (Jenkins *et al*, 1997; Male & May, 1997).

Epidemiology

Rates of violent and aggressive behaviour vary considerably across studies, ranging from 2% to 51% of those with intellectually disability population (Borthwick-Duffy, 1994; Emerson *et al*, 2001; Crocker *et al*, 2006). The differences in the prevalence of violence across studies were due to methodological variations that included factors such as study settings (e.g. institutional *v.* community), level of intellectual disability (profound intellectual disability to mild intellectual disability, as well as borderline intellectual disability), time-span surveyed (e.g. past month, past year or more) and age group (children, adolescents or adults) (McClintock *et al*, 2003).

Aetiology

Biological factors

Violent behaviour in people with intellectual disability can be driven by factors which also apply to those without intellectual disability (e.g. coexistent mental illness, substance misuse, certain personality disorders). Additional inherent factors arising from the intellectual disability such as poor regulation of frustration and anxiety can compound or act independently to trigger violent behaviour (Bhaumik et al, 2005).

Some specific biological factors which have been investigated with regard to their role in precipitating aggression in people with intellectual disability include epilepsy (Creaby et al, 1993), pain (Tenneij & Koot, 2008) and menstruation (Rodgers et al, 2006).

Psychosocial factors

People with intellectual disability are also more likely than the general population to be ascribed low social status and to encounter stigma from their peers (Crocker et al, 1998; Dovidio et al, 2000). In in-patient services, environmental factors such as overcrowding, high staff turnover and inadequate staff training may also contribute towards violent behaviour. Moreover, people with intellectual disability are more likely to be exposed to more severe forms of maltreatment. People with intellectual disability with a history of victimisation or abuse are at high risk of exhibiting violent behaviour (Strand et al, 2004). Gardener & Moffatt (1990) offered a multimodal explanation of aggression in people with intellectual disability that stressed the importance of individual setting conditions, environmental setting conditions, and maintaining factors.

A large national audit on the management of violence in in-patient services for people with intellectual disabilities conducted from 2001 to 2002 showed that aspects of the unit environment, such as noise, temperature and access to quiet spaces, had a significant impact on the risk of violence occurring. In addition, support being available for staff following a violent incident, good staff morale and good quality of communication to service users regarding their stay and treatment were found to be significantly positive factors (Deb & Roberts, 2005).

Assessment

All relevant biopsychosocial factors need to be explored in a multidisciplinary way. Functional assessment of behaviour is a commonly used process, with the aim to establish the relationship between behaviour and the function it serves for an individual. This is achieved by a process of data collection through observation of the trigger of the behaviour, identifying the behaviour itself, and identifying the consequence of the behaviour that continues to maintain it.

Risk assessment

It is important to recognise the need for evaluating the key domains of risk assessment and management that applies in the general population, but due consideration should also be given to biopsychosocial factors relevant in raising distress and anxiety in people with intellectual disability.

Objective violence risk assessment tools have been mostly validated in the offender population with intellectual disability. The Violence Risk Appraisal Guide (Quinsey *et al*, 1998), Historical Clinical Risk-20 (Webster *et al*, 1995), Short Dynamic Risk Scale (Quinsey *et al*, 2004) and Emotional Problem Scale (Prout & Strohmer, 1991) would appear to have some value in the evaluation of risk for future violent incidents when applied in high/ medium/low secure and community settings (Lindsay *et al*, 2008).

Prevention of violence in intellectual disability

Central to prevention of violence is a robust formulation of the biopsychosocial needs of an individual with intellectual disability and a comprehensive assessment of risk. Therapeutic consideration should be afforded to inherent factors of intellectual disability which lower the threshold for violence. These include poor problem-solving skills, impaired regulation of negative emotional experiences, reduced understanding of socially acceptable behaviour and empathic difficulties. A prevention care plan should be holistic and address all biological, psychological and social factors which may contribute to violent aggression in each individual.

One suggested way of minimising the impact of environment on behaviour is to train both staff and the patient to make the best use of the environment.

Management

It is essential that good-quality services are commissioned and provided to ensure that people with such additional and complex needs are appropriately cared for so that they can lead fulfilling lives in the community. Services should be local, provide individualised support, ensure innovative day opportunities and offer short breaks as respite for family carers.

Additional specialist services are required locally to support good mainstream practice as well as directly serve a small number of people with the most challenging needs. These services are usually found as part of a community learning disability team (Department of Health, 2007).

Interventions

Psychological interventions

Treatments based on psychological principles have strong empirical support (British Psychological Society, 2004).

Positive behaviour support

This is a person-centred approach to working with people with challenging behaviour. The aim is to replace problematic behaviour with functionally equivalent 'replacement' behaviours, while at the same time looking at the environmental and social factors that influence or maintain the behaviour, and increasing communication skills for the individual (Horner *et al*, 2002).

Cognitive–behavioural therapy (CBT)

There is randomised controlled trial evidence for the use of CBT in anger management in people with intellectual disability in both forensic secure and community settings (Willner, 2007). However, the use of CBT relies on language, which may reduce its utility in people with significant communication difficulties, and there have been no standardised approaches developed for its use in this population (Sturmey, 2004).

De-escalation

This is defined as the purposeful use of a complex range of communication and therapeutic intervention skills based on a knowledgeable understanding of the causes of violence and aggression. The aim is to prevent, reduce or manage the probability of violent or aggressive behaviour.

Medical interventions

Medical intervention for aggressive challenging behaviour can be effective where there is an underlying mental health or physical health problem which has been correctly diagnosed.

Psychotropic medication can also be used to attenuate some problems associated with violent behaviour where no medical/psychiatric cause is identified, but the evidence base for this is limited. A Cochrane review of antipsychotic medication for challenging behaviour confirmed that there is no randomised controlled trial-based information to suggest that antipsychotic medication is either helpful or harmful for adults with intellectual disability and challenging behaviour (Brylewski & Duggan, 2004). The more recent NACHBID (Neuroleptic for Aggressive CHallenging Behaviour in Intellectual Disability) randomised controlled trial also showed no significant benefits conferred by treatment with either risperidone or haloperidol in the treatment of aggressive challenging behaviour (Tyrer *et al*, 2008). This finding conflicts with the current situation where antipsychotic medication continues to be used in clinical practice for such purposes; Deb *et al* (2006) have produced a useful guide for the use of psychotropic medication in such cases. It is likely that psychotropic medication has some effect on the underlying anxiety and arousal state that are associated with an aggressive incident and therefore indirectly influence the manifestation of violence in a person.

Rapid tranquillisation

Most of the evidence for the use of rapid tranquillisation comes from studies among patients with psychiatric illnesses; therefore the inference drawn for its use among people who have intellectual disabilities has to be used with caution (Deb 7 Roberts, 2005).

Physical interventions

In the event of imminent violence, it may be necessary to use physical interventions. Wherever possible these should be detailed in an individual's care plan. There is a growing literature in this area, and the Department of Health (2002) and the British Institute of Learning Disabilities (2010) have published guidelines on this. Most studies in the UK support the notion that physical intervention should invoke no pain or very little pain in the patient who is being restrained. This proposal is supported by the finding that a high proportion of people who have intellectual disabilities have an altered pain threshold (Biersdorff, 1994). This, in combination with existing physical conditions such as heart or respiratory disease (conditions that are prevalent among people who have intellectual disabilities), contributes to the potential hazards associated with the physical restraint of a person with intellectual disability. The Mental Health Act 1983 *Code of Practice* states that physical intervention should be used 'as a last resort and never as a matter of course. It should be used proportionally in an emergency when there seems to be a real possibility that significant harm would occur if intervention is withheld' (Department of Health, 2008).

Legislation

The principles of the Mental Capacity Act 2005 and the Mental Health Act 1983 need to guide all assessment care and treatment decisions in this vulnerable patient population. This is discussed in more detail in Chapter 1.

References

Bhaumik, S., Nadkarni, S. S., Biswas, A. B., *et al* (2005) Service innovations: risk assessment in learning disability. *Psychiatric Bulletin*, **29**, 28–31.

Biersdorff, K. K. (1994) Incidence of significantly altered pain experience among individuals with developmental disabilities. *American Journal on Mental Retardation*, **98**, 619–631.

Borthwick-Duffy, S. A. (1994) Prevalence of destructive behaviors. A study of aggression, self-injury, and property destruction. In *Destructive Behavior in Developmental Disabilities: Diagnoses and Treatment* (eds T. Thompson & D. B. Gray), pp. 3–23. Sage.

British Institute of Learning Disabilities (2010) *BILD Code of Practice for the Use and Reduction of Restrictive Physical Interventions*. BILD.

British Psychological Society (2004) *Challenging Behaviours: Psychological Interventions for Severely Challenging Behaviours shown by People with Learning Disabilities*. BPS.

Brylewski, J. & Duggan, L. (2004) Antipsychotic medication for challenging behaviour in people with learning disability. *Cochrane Database of Systematic Reviews*, **3**, CD000377.

Creaby, M., Warner, M., Jamil, N., *et al* (1993) Ictal aggression in severely mentally handicapped people. *Irish Journal of Psychological Medicine*, **10**, 12–15.

Crocker, J., Major, B. & Steele, C. (1998) Social stigma. In *Handbook of Social Psychology* (eds D. T. Gilbert, S. Fiske & G. Lindzey), pp. 504–553. McGraw-Hill.

Crocker, A. G., Mercier, C., Lachapelle, Y., *et al* (2006) Prevalence and types of aggressive behaviour among adults with intellectual disabilities. *Journal of Intellectual Disability Research*, **50**, 652–661.

Deb, S. & Roberts, K. (2005) *The Evidence Base for the Management of Imminent Violence in Learning Disability Settings* (Occasional Paper OP57). Royal College of Psychiatrists.

Deb, S., Clarke, D. & Unwin, G. (2006) *Using Medication to Manage Behaviour Problems Among Adults with a Learning Disability: Quick Reference Guide*. University of Birmingham.

Department of Health (2002) *Guidance for Restrictive Physical Interventions: How to Provide Safe Services for People with Learning Disabilities and Autistic Spectrum Disorder*. Department of Health.

Department of Health (2007) *Services for People with Learning Disabilities and Challenging Behaviour or Mental Health Needs (Revised Edition)*. Department of Health.

Department of Health (2008) *Code of Practice: Mental Health Act 1983*. TSO (The Stationery Office).

Dovidio, J. F., Major, B. & Crocker, J. (2000) Stigma: introduction and overview. In *The Social Psychology of Stigma* (eds T. F. Heatherton, R. E. Kleck, M. R. Hebl, *et al*), pp. 1–30. Guilford Press.

Emerson, E., Kiernan, C., Alborz, A., *et al* (2001) The prevalence of challenging behaviors: a total population study. *Research in Developmental Disabilities*, **22**, 77–93.

Gardner, W. I. & Moffatt, C. (1990) Aggressive behaviour: definition, assessment, treatment. *International Review of Psychiatry*, **2**, 91–100.

Horner, R. H., Dunlap, G., Koegel, R. L., *et al* (2002) Positive behaviour support: evolution of an applied science. *Journal of Positive Behaviour Interventions*, **4**, 4–20.

Jenkins, R., Rose, J. & Lovell, C. (1997) Psychological well-being of staff working with people who have challenging behaviour. *Journal of Intellectual Disability Research*, **41**, 502–511.

Lindsay, W. R., Hogue, T. E., Taylor, J. L., *et al* (2008) Risk assessment in offenders with intellectual disability: a comparison across three levels of security. *International Journal of Offender Therapy and Comparative Criminology*, **52**, 90–111.

Male, D. B. & May, D. S. (1997) Burnout and workload in teachers of children with severe learning difficulties. *British Journal of Learning Disabilities*, **25**, 117–121.

McClintock, K., Hall, S. & Oliver, C. (2003) Risk markers associated with challenging behaviours in people with intellectual disabilities: a meta-analytic study. *Journal of Intellectual Disability Research*, **47**, 405–416.

Prout, T. H. & Strohmer, D. C. (1991) *Emotional Problem Scale*. Psychological Assessment Resources.

Quinsey, V. L., Book, A. & Skilling, T. A. (2004) A follow-up of deinstitutionalized men with intellectual disabilities and histories of antisocial behaviour. *Journal of Applied Research in Intellectual Disabilities*, **17**, 243–253.

Quinsey, V. L., Harris, G. T., Rice, M. E., *et al* (1998) *Violent Offenders: Appraising and Managing Risk*. American Psychological Association.

Rodgers, J., Lipscombe, J. & Santer, M. (2006) Menstrual problems experienced by women with learning disabilities. *Journal of Applied Research in Intellectual Disabilities*, **19**, 364–373.

Strand, M., Benzein, E. & Saveman, B. I. (2004) Violence in the care of adult persons with intellectual disabilities. *Journal of Clinical Nursing*, **13**, 506–514.

Sturmey, P. (2004) Cognitive therapy with people with intellectual disability: a selective review and critique. *Clinical Psychology and Psychotherapy*, **11**, 222–232.

Tenneij, N. H. & Koot, H. M. (2008) Incidence, types and characteristics of aggressive behaviour in treatment facilities for adults with mild intellectual disability and severe challenging behaviour. *Journal of Intellectual Disability Research*, **52**, 114–124.

Tyrer, P., Oliver-Africano, P. C., Ahmed, Z., *et al* (2008) Risperidone, haloperidol, and placebo in the treatment of aggressive hallenging behaviour in patients with intellectual disability: a randomised controlled trial. *Lancet*, **371**, 57–63.

Webster, C. D., Eaves, D., Douglas, K. S., *et al* (1995) *The HCR-20: The Assessment of Dangerousness and Risk*. Simon Fraser University & British Colombia Forensic Psychiatric Services Commission.

Willner, P. (2007) Cognitive behaviour therapy for people with learning disabilities: focus on anger. *Advances in Mental Health and Learning Disabilities*, **1**, 14–21.

CHAPTER 10

Management of violence in prisons

Ian Cumming

In addition to security, one of the core responsibilities of a prison is the management of violence. This is embodied within Prison Service Order PSI 64/2011, *Management of Prisoners at Risk of Harm to Self, to Others and from Others (Safer Custody)* (National Offender Management Service, 2012) (replacing PSO 2750, *Violence Reduction* (HM Prison Service, 2007)), which details the concept within a prison. It sets out a framework for 'delivering safer custody procedures and practices to ensure that prisons are safe places for all those who live and work there'. Perhaps in contrast to health services, its desired outcomes are to enable prisoners, staff and others feel safe and able to function effectively free from fear of violence, threatening behaviour, intimidation and bullying.

There is a national strategy which enables each prison to develop a local approach (or violence reduction strategy) within the resources available to them, and many prisons now have a violence reduction coordinator. Each establishment is required to have a strategy that incorporates the following:

- conflict resolution
- dynamic security
- effective risk management
- addressing organisational and environmental factors
- behaviour management for particular individuals
- offender management processes.

PSI 64/2011 states that each prison establishment is expected to have the capability (using the violence reduction toolkit) to develop a policy to reduce violence. Prisons are encouraged to adopt a problem-solving approach, based on collecting and analysing local data, formulating action plans and developing initiatives tailored to establishment needs. The focus is on a whole-prison approach, where 'all aspects of service delivery and prison life are considered as opportunities to create a safer environment' (HM Prison Service, 2007).

The Prison Service first defines violence with the starting point that certain levels can be tolerated or excused in any culture, but that toleration can lead to escalation. A common agreed threshold is, however, needed to allow others to report or challenge and apply appropriate sanctions.

It is to be noted that all staff who have contact with prisoners or carry out any form of assessment or management of prisoners, also have a responsibility for risk assessment and risk management.

The key aspects within the Prison Service are now discussed.

Reporting, recording and information-sharing

The Prison Service collates a large amount of information on offenders. Reporting is seen as a sign of a healthy environment and of confidence in the system and responses that come from it. There are many sources of information within a prison, such as security information reports as well as prisoner complaints forms.

Prevention is much higher on the prison agenda and it is to be noted that

'Every day, prison officers prevent dozens, perhaps hundreds of fights and assaults between prisoners. This remarkable achievement requires highly tuned interpersonal skills, but it isn't recognised or officially rewarded' (HM Prison Service, 2007).

Control and restraint in prisons

Historically and decades ago, the Prison Service had resolved situations through force of numbers, with the view that the more staff that were on hand, the more likely it was that a situation could be resolved without harm. The techniques and implementation strategy for control and restraint in prisons is relatively new and was not formally published as a manual until 1989. Prior to this, the Prison Service had utilised MUFTI (Minimum Use of Force Towards Inmates) training. A small group of staff were responsible for putting together the first control and restraint techniques and getting them recognised – 80% of these techniques are still in force today. The range of techniques has evolved to form the core manual on control and restraint that exists today (a restricted document with access limited to national control and restraint instructors and the Gold Command Suite). These techniques have been widely exported and learning has been shared with other agencies such as the police.

In 1988, the Prison Service opened the National Tactical Response Group, with six permanent members of staff; over the years the facility has evolved and now provides a range of environments (such as purpose-built cells) in which staff can practise techniques. There are also a range of other courses such as 'method of entry' and 'negotiating at height.'

In prisons, control and restraint is an essential part of prison officer training and is officially recognised by the Prison Service as the safest and most effective way of controlling concerted indiscipline across the estate.

97

Training of staff in the actual techniques of control and restraint can only be carried out by qualified control and restraint instructors. The techniques to be taught are detailed in a training manual.

The policy of force within prisons is enshrined within PSO1600, *Use of Force* (HM Prison Service, 2005); it details the circumstances in which force can be used and the framework for justifying the use of force. The use of force is only lawful if it is:

- reasonable
- proportionate
- necessary
- no more force than is necessary in the circumstances.

The policy document covers not only control and restraint techniques but also de-escalation skills, personal safety techniques and the use of batons. Practical techniques are detailed within the *Use of Force: Training Manual* (National Offender Management Service, 2006). The manual is issued in the form of a CD ROM to all governors and local control and restraint instructors. Staff using use-of-force techniques are nationally based and called 'Tornado response staff'.

Control and restraint techniques are used as a last resort in order to bring a violent or refractory prisoner under control. Techniques are used by a team of three officers, with the option of another person to control the legs, for as short a time as possible. Control and restraint techniques only use the force that is necessary to enable staff to cope competently and effectively with violent prisoners and potentially disruptive situations, with the minimum risk of injury to staff or prisoners.

Staff must continue to attempt to de-escalate the situation throughout the incident with the aim of releasing holds and locks, and must not employ control and restraint techniques when it is unnecessary to do so or in a manner which entails the use of more force than is necessary. The application of control and restraint holds may cause pain to a prisoner, and if the prisoner is compliant, the holds must be relaxed.

Incidents can roughly be demarcated into planned and unplanned. Planned incidents involving control and restraint are used when there is no urgency or immediate danger. In these situations, a supervisor will prepare staff for the incident and will notify a member of healthcare in advance, who should attend and observe the planned intervention. Unplanned incidents occur when there is an immediate threat to someone's life/limb or to the security of an establishment, and staff need to intervene straight away. In these situations a member of healthcare and a supervising officer will attend as soon as possible.

Where fewer than three officers are present (or in the case of multiple violent prisoners, a ratio of less than three officers to one violent prisoner) and it is necessary to use force immediately, staff will need to use whatever force is necessary to protect themselves and others – as long as such force is reasonable and proportionate in the circumstances as they see them.

All members of staff involved in the use of control and restraint (including the supervising officer) *must* complete a use of force form after each incident.

Searching in prisons

The National Offender Management Service's policy requires that in all prisons procedures are in place for the searching of prisoners, staff, domestic, official and professional visitors and contractors; these must be capable of detecting all items of contraband, including illegal substances. The procedures governing searching in prisons are laid out within the *National Security Framework* (National Offender Management Service, 2011). Searching is a key role of prisons and prison staff. Each prison has a searching strategy which will define the nature of the search and draw on risk assessments where appropriate. The searching strategy is agreed between prison management and the area manager or the director of high security if this is within a high-security prison.

Although the searching of staff will be carried out in all prisons on entry, the level and frequency of such searching at individual prisons is determined by local security and control needs and is set out in each prison's local searching strategy.

Visitors (official or otherwise) to prison will be familiar that searching is a potential issue and the guidance is such that visitors should expect this to take place with the level of searching depending on the category of prison. Searching is intended to detect contraband and other illegal activity. Illegal drugs and mobile telephones are the current priorities for the Prison Service. The Prison Service employs a variety of processes to enable detection such as use of CCTV, passive dogs and more recently BOSS – Bodily Orifice Security Scanner – on which individuals sit and which allows the detection of, for example, mobile telephones in bodily cavities.

Many prisons have dedicated search teams who regularly sweep and search a proportion of prisoners, although sometimes it is conducted on the basis of intelligence. These searches of cells are called 'fabric checks' and there has been some recent debate about their value. In some prisons, particularly some open prisons, a better use of resources may be achieved by carrying out only targeted, intelligence-led or random search programmes. Staff are also subject to searches, again often led by intelligence.

Prison officers carry out searches under The Prison Rules 1999, Rules 64 and 71, and in young offender prisons under The Young Offender Institution Rules 2000, Rules 69 and 70. Rule 41 of The Prison Rules is the main statutory provision governing when and how prisoners are to be searched and identifies three key principles:

1   Every prisoner shall be searched when taken into custody by an officer, on his reception into a prison and subsequently as the governor thinks necessary or as the Secretary of State may direct.

2   A prisoner shall be searched in as seemly a manner as is consistent with discovering anything concealed.

3   No prisoner shall be stripped and searched in the sight of another prisoner, or in the sight of a person of the opposite gender.

An officer may use reasonable force to affect the search (or not use force unnecessarily) and officers should not act deliberately in a manner calculated to provoke a prisoner. However, no more than an outer coat, jacket and gloves may be removed during a search without consent. Officers are themselves subject to searching as defined by Rule 64 of The Prison Rules. Only medical officers have the power to carry out intimate searches and only police officers have the power to carry out intimate searches of visitors or members of staff.

Prison officers also have powers of searching without consent when they suspect that an individual has a firearm, is carrying illegal drugs or is a danger to themselves or others.

Drug testing and detection in prisons

The presence of illegal drugs in prison is a constant challenge to all prisons in England and Wales and across the world. It is not just the effects of the drug use within prisons which is of consternation but the culture of debt, bullying and corruption which comes as a by-product.

It is an offence to use drugs or bring drugs into prisons. Before legislation had been introduced, visitors were normally either given a ban, put on closed visits or required to have mandatory searching (including strip searching) until they were no longer to be thought a risk. To update and introduce changes to the Prison Act 1952, from 1 April 2008 the penalties for smuggling contraband into a prison were strengthened and became an offence under Section 22 of the Offender Management Act 2007. The offence carries a penalty of up to 10 years and/or an unlimited fine.

Introduced in 1996, mandatory drug testing is one of the components of the Prison Service Drug Strategy (Ministry of Justice, 2006) to address the rising rate of drug misuse in prisons. Mandatory drug testing aims to:

- deter drug use in prison
- identify those to treat and those to punish
- provide information on the level of drug use and types of drugs used in prison.

In addition to drug testing on reception into a prison, drug testing is conducted on a random group of prisoners; all establishments are required to conduct tests on a fixed proportion of the population every month (between 5 and 10% of the population). Prisoners can also be tested if staff suspect that the prisoner has used drugs, and prisoners who have a history of drug misuse can also be selected for a frequent test programme.

It is recognised that mandatory drug testing can direct attention away from treatment and prevention and could also concentrate on what is considered a non-problem area, that of cannabis. There is also concern that the mandatory drug testing programme might cause prisoners to switch from cannabis to heroin because of the long time that cannabis remains in the urine. There have been further concerns about whether the use of mandatory drug testing has actually made any impact on drug use in prisons and that it is expensive and a poor indicator of drug use. A study by Edgar & O'Donnell (1998) indicated that a proportion of those known to use drugs in prison were not detected.

New initiatives were later introduced, including the increased use of passive dogs, voluntary testing programmes and key programmes such as CARAT (Counselling, Assessment, Referral, Advice and Throughcare).

To assess some of these issues, a major research project was undertaken in 2005 (Singleton *et al*, 2005). Based on a national study from 2001 which identified that 16% of prisoners were using illegal drugs in prison the week before interview (mainly cannabis and heroin), the study found that monthly mandatory drug tests correlated with prisoners' self-reported drug use but underestimated the level of self-reported misuse. Taking into account the differing detection times, it was felt that the mandatory drug test results for opiates indicated the frequency of use, whereas the self-report results for opiates reflected more closely to the numbers of users. It also showed that the use of cannabis in prisons had declined, whereas the use of heroin had remained fairly static; around 1% of prisoners had stopped using cannabis and had started using heroin.

Due to the high numbers of tests needed, prisons typically use 'on the spot' urine sticks which identify a range of drugs and their breakdown products. The Medicines and Healthcare products Regulatory Agency undertook a review of the analytical performance of these tests and found considerable variance in quality (Burtonwood, 2003). There is currently no mandatory regulation of drug testing services or test kit manufacturers. Some manufacturers comply voluntarily with an EU directive and additionally they can be prosecuted under the Consumer Protection Act 1987 and the Trade Descriptions Act 1968 if their products do not perform as intended.

References

Burtonwood, C. A. (2003) *Sixteen Devices for the Detection of Drugs of Abuse in Urine (MHRA Evaluation Report)*. Medicines and Healthcare products Regulatory Agency.

Edgar, K. & O'Donnell, I. (1998) *Mandatory Drug Testing in Prisons: The Relationship Between MDT and the Level and Nature of Drug Misuse* (Home Office Research Study 189). Home Office.

HM Prison Service (2005) *Use of Force* (Prison Service Order, No. 1600). HM Prison Service.

HM Prison Service (2007) *Violence Reduction* (Prison Service Order, No. 2750). HM Prison Service.

Ministry of Justice (2006) *10. Drug Strategy*. Ministry of Justice (http://www.justice.gov.uk/downloads/publications/hmps/2006/10001E7B10_drug_strategy_jul_06.pdf).

National Offender Management Service (2006) *Use of Force: Training Manual*. Ministry of Justice.

National Offender Management Service (2011) *National Security Framework 3.1: Searching The Person*. Ministry of Justice.

National Offender Management Service (2012) *Management of Prisoners at Risk of Harm to Self, to Others and from Others (Safer Custody)* (PSI 64/2011). Ministry of Justice (http://www.insidetime.org/resources/psi/psi-64-2011-safer-custody.pdf).

Singleton, N., Pendry, E., Simpson, T., *et al* (2005) *The Impact of Mandatory Drug Testing in Prisons*. Home Office.

CHAPTER 11

Liaison with the police, Crown Prosecution Service and MAPPA

Ruth McAllister

Offences committed by mental health patients

Police are regularly called to hospitals and community mental health sites when someone with a mental health problem commits a crime. In the past many offences, including violent offences, committed by mental health patients were neither investigated nor prosecuted. This was due to a perception that patients could not be held responsible for their actions, that the likelihood of conviction was unacceptably low or that prosecution was not necessary to protect the public if the patient was already in hospital. Modern police policy is that the criminal law has an equal application inside and outside mental health units and there should be a presumption that patients have the capacity in law to take responsibility for their actions. Mental health professionals should be prepared to liaise with the police and help them to make better-informed decisions about investigations. Positive action against the offender by the police may assist in future management of the patient.

The police should seek the views of the consultant in charge before deciding how best to deal with the matter. They may ask the consultant to assess whether the patient is fit to be interviewed and detained at a police station. This should be done as promptly as possible and the assessment forwarded in writing to the police custody officer, for the attention of the forensic medical examiner (police doctor) or custody nurse. The mental health trust should provide an appropriate adult to accompany the patient at police interview and ensure that they are legally represented.

If the patient is charged, the court may ask the consultant for a report on the patient's fitness to plead and stand trial. National Health Service staff should be prompt in responding to such requests and avoid passing them on to different teams and departments. Similarly, staff should cooperate with the police in arranging to provide witness statements and medical reports relating to the victim's injuries. Those who give statements should add their contact details and the dates when they know they will be unavailable to attend court, in order to avoid delay and additional court costs.

There may be occasions when immediate arrest is not possible or appropriate. This does not preclude prosecution at a later stage.

Clear guidelines should be available to staff and police, as in the example in Box 11.1. These should be discussed and agreed at local police liaison meetings.

The *Memorandum of Understanding between the Association of Chief Police Officers (ACPO) and the NHS Security Management Service* (NHS Security Management Service, 2004) provides a framework for the exchange of information between the police and mental health services. It sets out guidance to facilitate good working relationships and clear communication between all parties.

Part of the remit of the NHS Security Management Service is to support the work of the police in relation to assaults on staff and to the illegal use and supply of controlled drugs within the NHS. Its aim is primarily to protect NHS staff and resources rather than patients (Box 11.2). However, the NHS has a duty of care towards those who use its services and premises, particularly if they are young or vulnerable.

Box 11.1 Guidelines for staff and police when patients commit an offence

What the police will do

- Make contact and liaise with the senior person on duty (e.g. unit coordinator)
- Record and investigate any allegations
- Seek the views of the victim: if a victim of assault is unwilling or unable to substantiate an allegation, prosecution may still be appropriate if there are witnesses to the offence
- Seek the views of the consultant in charge
- Consider either arresting the suspect or issuing summons to court
- Give regular updates to the victim as to the progression of the case

What mental health unit staff will do

- Report offences to the police promptly
- Obtain a crime number
- Preserve the crime scene until police officers arrive
- Provide support and encouragement to the victim to prosecute
- The nurse in charge will ensure that all staff who are witnesses complete statements before the end of the shift

---

Box 11.2 Priorities of the NHS Security Management Service

- Tackling violence against staff and professionals working in the NHS
- Ensuring the security of property and assets
- Ensuring the security of drugs, prescription forms and hazardous materials
- Ensuring the security of maternity and paediatric wards

The *Memorandum of Understanding* (NHS Security Management Service, 2004) sets out guidance on the police response to incidents on NHS premises, including violence and drug- and alcohol-related incidents. It sets out the legal framework for cooperation and information-sharing and outlines a prosecution policy.

Principles guiding prosecution for assaults on NHS staff[1]

- The police will progress all cases of violence against NHS staff and will not formally caution assailants without obtaining the views of the victim.
- Violence against NHS staff is unacceptable; when it occurs while members of staff are undertaking their duties, it should be considered an aggravating factor as laid down by the Code for Crown Prosecutors (Crown Prosecution Service, 2013).
- It is essential that the case officer includes in the summary that the victim was on duty or that the incident was related to their role in the NHS. The impact of the offence on the resources available for NHS care (such as the need for replacement staff, or cancelled treatments because someone has been injured) should also be recorded in the case summary. Claims for compensation should be made to the court to demonstrate the financial costs.
- If continued contact between the assailant and the victim during the investigation might affect the prosecution process, the investigating officer must promptly notify the NHS health body and the clinical team must take appropriate action.

Where a police investigation is not taken forward for prosecution, the Legal Protection Unit of the NHS Security Management Service may instigate private criminal or civil proceedings.

When an offence is committed on NHS property, staff and police must cooperate to preserve evidence at the scene as far as possible.

Exchange of information between NHS and police

Regular meetings should take place between the police and the NHS health body and all serious incidents involving the police should be reviewed at these meetings. Staff should disclose urgent information to the police when it is in the public interest to do so, balancing the requirements of patient confidentiality with public protection needs. The police should disclose

---

1. Taken from NHS Security Management Service (2004) *Memorandum of Understanding between the Association of Chief Police Officers (ACPO) and the NHS Security Management Service*. NHS Security Management Service.

relevant information to the NHS health body: in some cases, they may have intelligence on an individual which is directly relevant to risk assessment (e.g. on behaviour during previous periods in custody) and should consider disclosing it. The exchange of information should be guided by written protocols, according to the principles set out in Box 11.3.

Disclosure of clinical information to the police should also be governed by the NHS code of practice on confidentiality (Department of Health, 2003: p. 34):

> 'Under common law, staff are permitted to disclose personal information in order to prevent and support detection, investigation and punishment of serious crime and/or to prevent abuse or serious harm to others where they judge, on a case by case basis, that the public good that would be achieved by the disclosure outweighs both the obligation of confidentiality to the individual patient concerned and the broader public interest in the provision of a confidential service.'

This clearly places an obligation on individual staff members to make a reasoned judgement about the balance of risk and benefit in each individual case when considering disclosure. There is no agreed definition of 'serious

---

Box 11.3 Guidance on information-sharing with the police

Personal data relating to clinical records can only be disclosed with the express written permission of the individual or by order of the courts.

Disclosure to the police may be exempt from the above requirement if the objective is:

- the prevention or detection of crime
- the apprehension or prosecution of offenders
- if failure to disclose would prejudice the objective.

Disclosure may be made only in respect of identified cases. Any police request for disclosure should make clear why the investigation or proceedings might fail without disclosure.

Personal information disclosed to the police:

- must be relevant
- must only be used for the purpose specified in the request.

If the information is found to be inaccurate, this must be notified to the data owner, who must correct it and notify all other recipients of the correction.

Information should be retained for the minimum period needed to achieve the stated objective, after which it must be returned or destroyed. It must be kept secure and access must be granted only to those with a duty to deal with it for the purpose of the disclosure request.

NHS Security Management Service (2004)

crime' but examples would include murder, manslaughter, rape and child abuse. The code of practice also gives a list of crimes that are not usually considered serious enough to warrant disclosure, such as theft, fraud and damage to property 'where financial loss is less substantial'.

Patients should be asked for consent to disclosure: if a decision is made to disclose without consent, the patient should be informed unless this would lead to an unacceptable increase in risk.

If there is doubt about whether disclosure without consent is justified, the consultant in charge or the Caldicott Guardian should be consulted.

The police may also make a formal request for information under the Data Protection Act 1998 or the Freedom of Information Act 2005.

Joint working protocols

Each NHS trust should have joint working protocols with the police force or forces that cover their area. The protocols should contain guidance on the management of issues where police and health service responsibilities overlap, such as:

- criminal activity in a healthcare setting
- information-sharing
- restraint
- search procedures
- Mental Health Act assessments (police support for community assessments and assessments of people in police custody)
- missing persons
- deaths in care and/or custody (for detained patients)
- serious incidents (hostage-taking, riot, major incidents requiring evacuation)
- handling drugs and hazardous substances
- surveillance
- infant abduction, where relevant
- press releases
- training and review.

The content of the protocols will vary from trust to trust. They need to be developed in cooperation with all the involved parties, including the primary care trust, acute trust, Social Services and ambulance services. Senior staff and front-line staff need to be represented.

Liaison with the Crown Prosecution Service

The consultant or another senior member of the clinical team should also consider liaison with the Crown Prosecution Service (CPS), which is the authority responsible for deciding the charge in all but the most minor cases. The CPS has undertaken to work with the police to ensure that a 'robust charging policy' is applied in cases of violence and abuse against NHS staff or vulnerable victims (Crown Prosecution Service, 2008). Medical information may alter the balance of decisions about where the public interest lies in such cases, for example, if prosecution of a patient who is already detained in hospital may reduce the risk of future violence by allowing consideration of a restriction order under the Mental Health Act 1983.

The CPS has stated that, in cases of verbal and physical assault against NHS staff, alcohol and drug misuse will not be regarded as valid mitigating factors but rather as aggravating features. Charging standards provide for a charge of assault occasioning actual bodily harm when aggravating features are present, even if the injuries suffered are more typical of common assault. Psychological harm is included in the concept of actual bodily harm.

Diversion from prosecution

It may be in the interests of the victim, the wider community and the suspect to consider alternatives to the formal court process. These include caution, which may be simple or conditional. In a conditional caution, the offender must comply with conditions which may be aimed at rehabilitation or reparation, or may impose restrictions. If the offender fails to comply, they may be prosecuted for the original offence. Offences with aggravating features will not normally be considered suitable for a caution and the police have agreed not to caution offenders for assaults on staff without obtaining the views of the victim (NHS Security Management Service, 2004). Simple caution does not preclude private prosecution or civil action against an assailant.

Disagreements about charging decisions should be raised with the NHS Security Management Service liaison officer.

Mentally disordered offenders

The guidance issued by the NHS Security Management Service on reporting assaults against NHS staff to the police (NHS Security Management Service, 2003) contains a confused passage suggesting that assaults should be reported only 'if staff present have formed an initial view that the offender's behaviour has not arisen as a result of any condition or treatment' (Crown Prosecution Service, 2008). On the other hand, 'significant mental or physical ill health' is a factor against prosecution unless the offence is serious and/or there is a real possibility that it may be repeated. Even if violent behaviour towards staff is directly motivated by delusions, this should not necessarily be a factor against prosecution. Prosecution may occasionally be helpful in management, for example by allowing consideration of a restriction order under Section 41 of the Mental Health Act.

In making its charging decisions, the CPS will consider:

- whether the offender is already receiving treatment which the court might order on conviction
- the suspect's legal status in hospital (i.e. whether informal or detained)
- the seriousness and persistence of the violent or abusive behaviour
- the views of the victim(s)
- the suspect's fitness to be arrested, detained, interviewed and charged, and their fitness to plead.

Prosecutors may consider applying for community punishments and may seek help from NHS staff in drafting appropriate conditions. Prohibited activity or exclusion requirements under the Criminal Justice Act 2003, or a restraining order under the Protection from Harassment Act 1997 may be used to restrict unwanted conduct and to protect victims. Cooperation with health staff is needed to ensure that the conditions offer protection to the victim without excluding the offender from essential services.

The *Memorandum of Understanding* (Crown Prosecution Service, 2008) sets out the responsibilities of the CPS to victims and witnesses, which include:

- providing a single point of contact
- informing victims and witnesses of decisions
- notifying victims and witnesses of hearings and of the need to give evidence
- notifying victims and witnesses of outcomes
- providing special measures for vulnerable witnesses or those subject to intimidation
- ensuring that prosecutors have the necessary information to allow the court to make a compensation order if appropriate
- ensuring that prosecutors have a current victim impact statement.

Multi-Agency Public Protection Arrangements (MAPPA)

The Criminal Justice Act 2003 requires local criminal justice agencies to work in partnership with other bodies who deal with violent and sexual offenders, to protect the public from serious harm. Police, prison and probation services have a statutory duty to set up and chair administrative arrangements so that the agencies involved with such offenders can coordinate their efforts. Other agencies, such as health, housing, job centres, victim liaison and Social Services departments, have a duty to cooperate and share information. The relevant information is stored on a central database known as ViSOR (Violent and Sex Offender Register), which is managed by the police. A MAPPA is not, therefore, a legal entity in itself but a set of arrangements to coordinate partnership-working.

It is an important principle of the MAPPA process that each of the cooperating agencies retains its full responsibility and obligations towards the offender, which cannot be overridden by the MAPPA process. Current guidance (National Offender Management Service, 2012) explicitly states that:

> '[...]no agency should feel pressured to agree to a course of action which they consider is in conflict with their statutory obligations and wider responsibility for public protection.' (p. 1)

> 'While consensus may be reached and joint action agreed, they remain the responsibility of each agency. MAPPA does not aggregate the responsibility and authority of the agencies involved. Instead it clarifies the role each agency is to play.' (p. 11)

In practice, this means that, although health services must cooperate with the MAPPA process to allow effective liaison with other agencies, MAPPA should not override clinical judgement or dictate decisions. Disclosure of personal information about the patient should be limited to what is directly relevant to the risk management process (not wholesale copying of exhaustive reports) and, if electronic, must be by secure email.

Multi-Agency Public Protection Arrangements deal with registered sex offenders under the Sex Offenders Act 2007; violent offenders who have received a custodial sentence of greater than 12 months or its equivalent; and any other offender who, because of features of the offence, poses a risk of serious harm to the public.

Multi-Agency Public Protection Arrangement activity is organised into three levels of involvement. At level 1, the risk is managed by a single agency and MAPPA monitors progress. At level 2, the active involvement of more than one agency is required. Level 2 offenders are monitored at meetings of senior representatives from the participating agencies: for mental health this should be at consultant level. Level 3 is reserved for a few offenders who pose a high or very high risk of harm, which can only be managed at a senior level, or where there is exceptional public interest and a potential threat to public confidence in the criminal justice system.

In practice, most mentally disordered offenders who are eligible for MAPPA can be managed at Level 1, because the need for public protection can be met within the framework of the care programme approach process, mental health review tribunal and conditional discharge. Where there are specific difficulties, such as discharge by a tribunal against professional advice, non-compliance with the care programme approach or continued criminal activity such as drug dealing, it is appropriate to refer to MAPPA level 2.

Multi-Agency Public Protection Arrangements also has a duty to report on its activity and work with lay advisors. In each area there is a strategic management board for MAPPA, on which there should be senior mental health representation; some areas also have a mental health advisory group.

References

Crown Prosecution Service (2008) Memorandum of Understanding between the NHS Counter Fraud and Security Management Service and the Crown Prosecution Service. Available at: http://www.cps.gov.uk/publications/agencies/mounhs.html.

Crown Prosecution Service (2013) *The Code for Crown Prosecutors*. CPS.

Department of Health (2003) *Confidentiality: NHS Code of Practice*. Department of Health.

National Offender Management Service (2012) *MAPPA Guidance 2012. Version 4*. Ministry of Justice.

NHS Security Management Service (2003) *Tackling Violence Against Staff. Explanatory Notes for Reporting Procedures Introduced by Secretary of State Directions in November 2003* (updated June 2009). NHS Security Management Service.

NHS Security Management Service (2004) *Memorandum of Understanding between the Association of Chief Police Officers (ACPO) and the NHS Security Management Service*. NHS Security Management Service.

CHAPTER 12

Information-sharing with victims of crime committed by persons with mental disorders

Miriam Barrett and Dominic Beer

As a general rule, a patient's treatment and progress in hospital are confidential and, unless the patient consents to information being shared, this limits the information that can be disclosed, for example about an offender's release (Department of Health, 2003).

Under the 2007 amendments of the Mental Health Act 1983, victims had their rights extended to being able to give their views about conditions which might be attached to offenders either being conditionally discharged or being considered for discharge under SCT.

The local probation board retains responsibility for liaising with the victim concerned. Further information regarding responsibilities for clinical staff who work with this group of patients – either in the NHS or the independent sector – can be found in guidance on the extension of victims' rights under the Domestic Violence, Crime and Victims Act 2004 (Department of Health, 2008a).

Appendix I lists the support groups that victims of crime can contact.

Mental Health Act 1983 Code of Practice

The Mental Health Act 1983 *Code of Practice* (Department of Health, 2008b: p. 151) provides guidance on information for victims of crimes. According to this guidance, people who are victims of certain mentally disordered offenders detained in hospital now have rights under the Domestic Violence, Crime and Victims Act 2004 (Sections 35–45) to make representations and receive information about that patient's discharge.

This places a number of duties on hospital managers in relation to certain unrestricted patients detained under Part III, who have committed sexual or violent crimes. One of these duties is to liaise with victims in order to inform them whether the patient's discharge is being considered, whether the patient is to move to SCT and of any conditions on the CTO relating to contact with the victim and their family. Other duties include forwarding representations made by victims to people responsible for making decisions on discharge or SCT.

In other circumstances, concerning crimes of a different and not a sexual or violent nature, professionals should encourage (but cannot require) mentally disordered offender patients to agree to share information that will allow victims and their families to be informed of their progress. This may have the benefit of reducing the danger of harmful confrontations after a discharge of which victims were unaware.

Domestic Violence, Crime and Victims Act 2004

The Domestic Violence, Crime and Victims Act 2004 is concerned with criminal justice and concentrates on legal protection and assistance to victims of crime, particularly domestic violence. Its purpose is to ensure that victims of particular crimes are able to express their views about both the sentencing and release of the offender concerned.

The offences covered in the Act which apply to those convicted or to those dealt with using a hospital order or restriction order include:

- murder or an offence specified in Schedule 15 to the Criminal Justice Act 2003;
- an offence in respect of which the patient or offender is subject to the notification requirements of Part II of the Sexual Offences Act 2003;
- an offence against a child within the meaning of Part 2 of the Criminal Justice and Court Services Act 2000.

The requirements apply when an offender has been convicted of sexual or violent crimes or where a person has been charged with those offences, found not guilty by reason of insanity and as a result a hospital order is made.

The Domestic Violence, Crime and Victims Act requires the local probation board to seek victims' views about any conditions to be attached to a proposed transfer direction or restriction direction.

Role and responsibilities of the probation board

England and Wales

The probation board has the responsibility to ensure that a victim can make representations to a court about the need to consider whether the offender or patient should be subject to licence or supervised restrictions on release and, if so, what those conditions should be.

These representations should be considered by the court or mental health review tribunal at the time of release or conditional discharge. They have no legal force until the court or tribunal makes an order and the patient is entitled to contest them.

The probation board is also responsible for ensuring that victims receive information about any conditions or restrictions placed on an offender or patient.

113

The Home Office must inform the probation board of any intention by the Home Secretary to change, lift or discharge any restrictions of any hospital orders, hospital directions and transfer directions as defined in Sections 37(4), 42(1), 42(2), 45(3)(a) and (b), 47(1) and 49(2) of the Mental Health Act.

Mental health review tribunals must inform the relevant probation board if an application is made to the tribunal by a patient under Sections 69, 70 or 75 of the Mental Health Act, or if the Secretary of State refers the patient's case to the tribunal under Section 71 of the Act.

Scotland and Northern Ireland

Similar duties, rights and responsibilities are described in the Justice (Northern Ireland) Act 2002.

The Victim Notification Scheme in Scotland applies to people convicted of a crime and not those disposed of by a court using the Mental Health (Care and Treatment) (Scotland) Act 2003.

Further reading

Ministry of Justice (2009) *Duties to Victims under the Domestic Violence, Crime and Victims Acts 2004: Guidance for Clinicians.* TSO (The Stationery Office).

Office for Criminal Justice Reform (2005) *The Code of Practice for Victims of Crime.* Criminal Justice System.

Victims of Crime Office (2010) *Victims Charter and Guide to the Criminal Justice System.* Department of Justice and Law Reform.

References

Department of Health (2003) *Confidentiality: NHS Code of Practice.* Department of Health.

Department of Health (2008a) *Mental Health Act 2007: Guidance on the Extension of Victims' Rights under the Domestic Violence, Crime and Victims Act 2004.* Ministry of Justice.

Department of Health (2008b) *Code of Practice: Mental Health Act 1983.* TSO (The Stationery Office).

CHAPTER 13

Clinical governance

Dominic Beer and Sachin Patel

By law, all hospitals in England are responsible for making sure that the care and treatment they provide meet government standards of quality and safety (Care Quality Commission, 2013). Through the systematic approach of clinical governance, these standards can be met and developed alongside improving the overall care provided by organisations.

In relation to the management of violence, the core elements of training and education, audit, research and development, openness, risk management and information management can be applied. These include the provision of adequate training in risk management, ensuring processes of recording untoward incidents, transparency in reporting incidents, use of evidence-based management of violence and auditing practice to ensure basic standards are met. Through this fluid, progressive approach, organisations can provide the best quality management of violence in the clinical setting.

Core standards

The Department of Health (2004) has set out common objective standards which apply across all NHS organisations. Among the core standards, a selection is relevant in providing quality management of violence. These are included in the domains of safety, clinical and cost effectiveness, governance, and care environment and amenities.

Safety

Core standard C1 stipulates:

Health care organisations protect patients through systems that

(a) identify and learn from all patient safety incidents and other reportable incidents, and make improvements in practice based on local and national experience and information derived from the analysis of incidents; and

(b) ensure that patient safety notices, alerts and other communications concerning patient safety which require action are acted upon within required time-scales.

Healthcare organisations should therefore have a defined reporting process at a local level. The National Patient Safety Agency provides guidance on the process and standards of data-reporting via the reporting and learning system (National Reporting and Learning Service, 2009). Reported incidents are analysed to identify root causes and likelihood of repetition. Through learning from untoward incidents, the NHS is able to promote patient safety through harnessing learning; it becomes an organisation with a memory (Department of Health, 2001).

Clinical and cost effectiveness

Core standard C5(a) stipulates:

> Health care organisations ensure that they conform to NICE technology appraisals and, where it is available, take into account nationally agreed guidance when planning and delivering treatment and care.

Therefore healthcare organisations must take into account when planning and delivering care, nationally agreed best practice as defined in national service frameworks, NICE clinical guidelines (National Institute for Health and Clinical Excellence, 2005) and other nationally agreed guidance. Clinicians should be involved in prioritising, conducting, reporting and acting on clinical audits. They will also contribute by reviewing the effectiveness of clinical services through evaluation, audit or research.

Governance

Core standard C11 stipulates:

> Health care organisations ensure that staff concerned with all aspects of the provision of health care
> (a) are appropriately recruited, trained and qualified for the work they undertake;
> (b) participate in mandatory training programmes; and
> (c) participate in further professional and occupational development commensurate with their work throughout their working lives.

Local organisations must provide training specific to the management of violence prior to working and refresher courses to ensure safe working practices. The NHS Security Management Service has published a syllabus, setting out minimum standards for training of all staff working in mental healthcare settings (NHS Security and Management Service, 2005).

Care environment and amenities

Core standard C20(a) stipulates:

> Health care services are provided in environments which promote effective care and optimise health outcomes by being a safe and secure environment which protects patients, staff, visitors and their property, and the physical assets of the organisation.

Healthcare organisations should aim to minimise the health, safety and environmental risks to patients, staff and visitors, in accordance with NHS occupational health and safety standards (Partnership for Occupational Safety and Health in Healthcare, 2010).

Care Quality Commission

In the UK, the Care Quality Commission ensures that healthcare providers meet acceptable government-set standards of care. Within the 28 essential outcomes when assessing standards of quality and safety (Care Quality Commission, 2010), the list below is pertinent when considering the management of violence in mental healthcare settings.

- *Outcome 4: Care and welfare of people who use services* – People should get safe and appropriate care that meets their needs and supports their rights.
- *Outcome 7: Safeguarding people who use services from abuse* – People should be protected from abuse and staff should respect their human rights.
- *Outcome 9: Management of medicines* – People should be given the medicines they need when they need them, and in a safe way.
- *Outcome 10: Safety and suitability of premises* – People should be cared for in safe and accessible surroundings that support their health and welfare.
- *Outcome 12: Requirements relating to workers* – People should be cared for by staff who are properly qualified and able to do their job.
- *Outcome 13: Staffing* – There should be enough members of staff to keep people safe and meet their health and welfare needs.
- *Outcome 16: Assessing and monitoring the quality of service provision* – The service should have quality checking systems to manage risks and assure the health, welfare and safety of people who receive care.
- *Outcome 21: Records* – People's personal records, including medical records, should be accurate and kept safe and confidential.

Guidance of acceptable standards is provided in detail by the Care Quality Commission. In terms of the management of violence, areas to be considered include providing a safe environment, procedures for assessing and minimising risk, safe use of rapid tranquillisation, ensuring staff are suitably trained, ensuring systems for reporting incidents are in place and that organisations monitor and improve the quality of services provided.

Audit

The National Institute for Health and Clinical Excellence (2005) produce audit criteria in their guidelines based on the key priorities for simple implementation.

Royal College of Psychiatrists' National Audit of Violence

On behalf of the Healthcare Commission, the National Collaborating Centre for Nursing and Supportive Care has liaised closely with the audit team at the Royal College of Psychiatrists, and has devised audit tools and conducted an audit on the short-term management of violence in psychiatric in-patient settings (Royal College of Psychiatrists' Centre for Quality Improvement, 2007a,b).

In addition to setting audit standards by consensus opinion (Royal College of Psychiatrists' Centre for Quality Improvement, 2007c), a tool is provided via three modules covering various aspects of the management of violence (www.rcpsych.ac.uk/crtu/centreforqualityimprovement/nationalauditofviolence.aspx). These include questionnaire screening of staff, service users and visitors, an environmental audit and a review of violent incidents including case-note reviews of rapid tranquillisation.

Quality improvement tools

The Healthcare Quality Improvement Partnership has published new guidance on the use of quality improvement tools that can be applied through clinical audit to improve services (Dixon & Pearce, 2011). The process of audit has been developed and redefined over the years to focus on quality improvement. Various quality improvement tools can be used to assist the process of audit at specific stages. This is designed to bring about immediate, positive changes in the delivery of healthcare in specific settings.

Summary

- Core standards for basic care are set by the Department of Health and must be met by mental healthcare organisations.
- Care Quality Commission inspections will assess various aspects of the management of violence in local organisations to ensure standards are met.
- Good-quality management of violence can be provided in organisations which have governance systems in place.
- There are many aspects of the management of violence which can be audited. Quality improvement tools can be used to bring about more immediate, positive changes to healthcare.

References

Care Quality Commission (2010) Essential Standards of Quality and Safety. CQC.
Care Quality Commission (2013) What Standards you have a Right to Expect from the Regulation of your Hospital. CQC.
Department of Health (2001) Building a Safer NHS: Implementing an Organisation with a Memory. TSO (The Stationery Office).

Department of Health (2004) *Standards for Better Health* (updated 2006). Department of Health.

Dixon, N. & Pearce, M. (2011) *Guide to Using Quality Improvement Tools to Drive Clinical Audits*. Healthcare Quality Improvement Partnership.

National Institute for Health and Clinical Excellence (2005) *The Short-term Management of Disturbed/Violent Behaviour in In-patient Psychiatric Settings and Emergency Departments* (Clinical Guideline CG25). NICE.

National Reporting and Learning Service (2009) *Data Quality Standards: Guidance for Organisations Reporting to the Reporting and Learning System (RLS)*. National Patient Safety Agency.

NHS Security and Management Service (2005) *Promoting Safe and Therapeutic Services*. NHS Security and Management Services.

Partnership for Occupational Safety and Health in Healthcare (2010) *Occupational Health and Safety Standards*. NHS Employers.

Royal College of Psychiatrists' Centre for Quality Improvement (2007a) *Healthcare Commission National Audit of Violence 2006–7: Final Report – Working Age Adult Services*. Healthcare Commission.

Royal College of Psychiatrists' Centre for Quality Improvement (2007b) *Healthcare Commission National Audit of Violence 2006–7: Final Report – Older People's Services*. Healthcare Commission.

Royal College of Psychiatrists' Centre for Quality Improvement (2007c) *National Audit of Violence: Standards for In-patient Mental Health Services*. Healthcare Commission.

Appendix: Organisations that victims of crime can contact

General

Home Office
www.gov.uk
Help and support for victims of crime.

Police community safety units
http://content.met.police.uk/Site/communitysafetyunit
Every London borough has a team of specially trained officers whose task is to investigate crimes such as domestic violence or if someone is targeted because of their race, faith, sexual orientation or disability. This website provides more information and advises on how to get in touch with your local community safety unit.

Charities

Crime Concern
www.crimeconcernuk.net
A national crime reduction charity which runs more than 60 projects across England and Wales, many of which are youth and neighbourhood-focused, as well as providing information on services, projects and how to become a volunteer.

Rape Crisis Federation
www.rapecrisis.org.uk
National voice for female survivors of sexual violence and abuse, provides facilities and resources to support rape crisis groups throughout England and Wales.

Refuge
www.refuge.org.uk
Refuge's network of safe houses provides emergency accommodation for women and children fleeing abuse. They offer emotional support and practical information.

Rights of Women
www.rightsofwomen.org.uk
Free legal advice on sexual violence, domestic violence, trafficking, child sex offences and family-related sex offences.

Survivors UK
www.survivorsuk.org
Supports and provides resources for men who have experienced any form of sexual violence.

Victim Support
www.victimsupport.org.uk
National independent charity for people affected by crime, supports victims by providing advice and promoting the rights of victims and witnesses in all aspects of criminal justice and social policy.

Women's Aid
www.womensaid.org.uk
National charity working to end domestic violence against women and children. It supports a network of over 500 domestic and sexual violence services across the UK.

Support agencies

Domestic violence

All Wales Domestic Abuse and Sexual Violence Helpline
www.allwaleshelpline.org.uk
Tel: 0808 80 10 800

Men's Advice Line
www.mensadviceline.org.uk
Tel: 0808 801 0327

National Domestic Violence Helpline
www.nationaldomesticviolencehelpline.org.uk
Tel: 0808 2000 247

Republic of Ireland Domestic Abuse Helpline
www.womensaid.ie
Tel: 1800 341 900

Respect
For domestic violence perpetrators.
www.respect.uk.net
Tel: 0808 802 40 40

Scotland Domestic Abuse Helpline
www.scottishdomesticabusehelpline.org.uk
Tel: 0800 027 1234

Women's Aid Federation Northern Ireland
www.womensaidni.org
Tel: 0800 917 1414

Other

Broken Rainbow UK
www.brokenrainbow.org.uk
Tel: 0300 999 5428

NSPCC
www.nspcc.org.uk
Tel: 0808 800 500

National Offender Management Service (NOMS) Victim Helpline
If a prisoner contacts you and you do not want this to happen again, or if you have any concerns about possible release, you can use a phone helpline to make sure that the prison governor knows your concerns.
Tel: 0845 758 5112

Support for women and children from multicultural backgrounds

Apna Ghar Housing Association
Housing support for people with disabilities
www.agha.org.uk
Tel: 020 8795 5405

Black Association of Women Step Out
www.bawso.org.uk
Tel: 0800 731 8147

Chinese Information and Advice Centre
www.ciac.co.uk
Tel: 020 7734 1039

Foreign and Commonwealth Office
www.fco.gov.uk
Tel: 020 7008 1500

Jewish Women's Aid Helpline
www.jwa.org.uk
Tel: 0808 801 0500

The Kiran Project
www.kiranproject.org.uk
Tel: 020 8558 1986

Muslim Community Helpline
http://muslimcommunityhelpline.org.uk
Tel: 020 8904 8193/020 8908 6715

Somalian Women's Centre
Tel: 020 8752 1787

Southall Black Sisters
www.southallblacksisters.org.uk
Tel: 020 8571 9595/020 8571 0800

Turkish Cypriot Women's Project
www.tcwp.org.uk
Tel: 0208 340 3300

Index

Compiled by Liza Furnival

Page numbers in *italics* refer to figures or boxes